JOB LOSS, STAGE 7 CANCER, AND 14 MONTHS OF CHEMOTHERAPY COULD NOT BREAK SUE MARTIN'S POSITIVE SPIRIT. THIS IS HER INSPIRATIONAL SURVIVAL STORY.

I Shed Two Tears and kicked it with attitude is an inspiring true story of surviving and thriving cancer during the Great Recession. Job loss, stage three cancer, 14 months of chemotherapy, while navigating a new job, were challenges, not obstacles. Sue Martin not only survived, but she also thrived in her new environment and beat all of the odds stacked against her. A healthy dose of laughter and positive thinking were the keys to success. This is a story of never giving up, and always seeing the bright side to moving forward. Excellent pearls of wisdom for crisis survival.

Praise for I Shed Two Tears

"Sue is a remarkable lady who inspired me from the moment she shared her story...I will be one of the first to read her book as I know it will be filled with brilliance on how to beat cancer with a positive outlook surrounded by humor and passion for life."—*Phil Molyneux, former President and COO, Sony Electronics*

"... Everyone who reads *I Shed Two Tears* will come out the better. It is not only for those who are currently in the fight of their life, but also for their caregivers. So much insight to be learned by us all...."—*Shaunna Tafelski*

"Sue Martin was my patient...She accepted her diagnosis with a positive attitude and jumped on board to focus on her treatment plan. Sue moved forward with life by starting a new job just weeks after her mastectomy."—*Dr. Jyoti Arya, M.D., Reconstructive Surgeon*

"Brave: adj. /brāv/ ready to face and endure danger or pain; showing courage. Synonyms: valiant, heroic, lionhearted, bold, fearless, gallant, courageous, undaunted, Sue Martin..."—*Donna Johnson*

Excerpt

After thoroughly explaining the extensive list of upcoming medical procedures from mastectomy, to chemo, to radiation, and finally reconstruction, Dr. Kurtzhals routinely inquired "Do you have any questions for me?"

"Yes, how soon after the mastectomy can I go back to work?"

She laughed and said "With your attitude, five to seven days. The poor woman who just left my office was sobbing and wanted 20-22 weeks off from work. She's going to have a very long road ahead of her."

"Great, because I had an interview a week ago and I feel pretty confident about it. If they offer me the job, I want to start working as soon as possible."

Yes, I will kick it with my attitude, I thought to myself. She assured me that my approach would ensure a technical knockout with several rounds of chemo cocktails and a few weeks at the tanning salon, my pet name for the radiation lab. For me, joking about the plethora of treatments, kept my spirits up. My laughter put people at ease, and put their tears at bay-- most of the time.

I Shed Two Tears

Sue Martin

Moonshine Cove Publishing, LLC

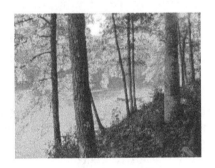

Abbeville, South Carolina
U.S.A.

First Moonshine Cove edition
2021

ISBN: 9781952439179

Library of Congress LCCN: 2021907820

© Copyright 2021 by Sue Martin

Cover images public domain; cover and interior design by Moonshine Cove staff

For Tanya, forever an angel in heaven.

About the Author

Sue Martin is a retired marketing professional with a BS in Business from SDSU, a BA in Humor from the

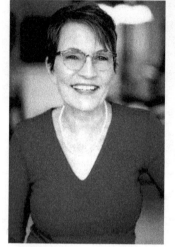

Cancer Survivor School of Life, and an MA in Creativity from her mother's DNA. She's a firm believer in tackling life's unexpected challenges with her funny bone. Job loss, the Great Recession, and cancer were slain with laughter.

http://www.ishedtwotears.com

Preface

When I was diagnosed with Stage 3 breast cancer, I decided early on that the best way to keep family and friends updated would be to write a blog.

I decided from the get-go that I would use my zany sense of humor to joke about all my procedures. I detailed my appointments, treatments, reactions and everyday life of battling cancer. I was very open and honest. In many cases, especially with my brothers, I would give them too much information (TMI). I loved teasing them and making them squirm.

I had pet names for treatments such as happy hour for chemo cocktails, tanning salon at the spa, made up names of characters who did not play nice, and used real names of those who did.

Over the course of 14 months of treatment and blogging, I had many friends encourage me to write a book. I knew I would do it, but little things like employment, art, quilting, and sculpting got in the way.

But the people who really encouraged me to finish writing and publishing it were the many cancer patients I spoke with to steer them off the cliff of doom and gloom and onto the positive path to fight with passion and humor. One of my favorite new cancer sisters was the delightful Shaunna Tafelski, whose brother-in-law is my ex-brother-in-law.

We never met in person, but we hit it off right away. We're both crafty and had both joined the breast cancer sisterhood, not by choice. When she was diagnosed, she was frightened, as any mother of teenage sons would be. My sister's ex-husband, Charlie, was her sister's husband, and he reached out to Sandra to see if I would to talk to Shaunna about beating cancer, and of course I did.

We were chatting in Facebook for over an hour, when I suggested she give me a call. It was much easier talking live and she could snowball me with her abundant questions. Our phone conversation lasted over three hours.

I told her that the coolest and most empowering thing I did was to have my portrait taken when I was bald. At first, she was shocked and said she didn't think she could do it. My positive attitude and my joking and laughing with her was contagious. I actually convinced her to have her photo taken bald. She is so stunning in her photo and you can see the determination to survive in her eyes. Check out her many talents and creativity on her blog www.temptingthyme.com.

There were many other cancer patients who I was able to convince to fight with determination and a sense of humor. I told them without hope, you cannot win. Several eventually lost their battle, but there were many who successfully slayed their own cancer beast.

Retirement has given me the quiet time needed to reflect and finish writing my book, in order to share my journey of beating cancer. I hope it will inspire others to fight the fight with strength, determination, and a ginormous dose of laughter. I also hope that friends and family of those with cancer, can find the strength to lift up their loved one to be positive throughout their private journey. You can do this!

Acknowledgment

I first of all want to thank all my family and friends for putting up with my relentless request of no tears, no crying, and no pity parties. I was pretty brutal on you, but I truly needed to maintain my upbeat attitude to get through the entire journey and successfully remain above dirt. It worked out fabulously.

Huge thanks to my immediate family my husband Denny and sons Tyler and Kyle, for not only not crying in front of me, but also for driving me home from some of my treatments. Huge thanks to my sister, Sandra for coming with me to chemo to have creative fun with our crafting projects, and especially to keep me laughing. My brothers Scott, Rob, and Jerry, who put up with my TMI banter about breast lopping and replacement parts. Thanks to Mom for not crying on the phone, when I broke the news to her.

My great support team, who came out to do the Breakaway Mile at the Amgen tour of California. Denny, Scott, Vienna, Sandra, Sara, Adam, and Boyd. Friends, Donna, Jenn, John, Jordyn, Christina, Jamal, Djoser, Asiya, Taharqa, Pat, Gordon, Matt, Jennifer, Reg, and Joy also joined us for the day.

I want to thank all of you who were early readers and offered feedback starting with, Pamela Corsentino, Veronica Glickman, Regina Hunter, Pam Homan, Roseanne Gendreau, Diana Loewiski, Patricia Ray, Camille Akin, Laurie Dooley, and Christina Burruss.

I am so thankful for my marvelous medical team who led me through the murky waters to cancer freedom, Dr. Pamela Kurtzhals, Dr. Joan Kroener, Dr. Ray Lin, Dr. Jyoti Arya, Dr. Allison Estabrook, Dr Julie Barone, and the fabulous Patti Joyce for her creative wig that allowed me to go incognito at my new job.

Foreword

In 2001, Destiny's Child had a smash hit album and title song, named *Survivor*. The band's video showed the trio "surviving" a shipwreck on an island and then "fighting" to stay alive. Do you have a visual? Is the tune in your head? If not, Google it. Once you listen to the song, the fierce lyrics, the upbeat tempo, the women's attitude, you'll know why Sue Martin comes to my mind. Every time I hear this song. I think of my friend, Sue "The Survivor" Martin.

You see Sue is no ordinary gal. She is not a super-hero with special powers. But she does possess an inner fight and an uncanny ability to approach any task with a warrior-like quality. Her story is extraordinary. It's real. It's raw. It's a whole lotta 'tude. This book is Sue's "kick-it-in-the-pants" day-by-day experience with her battle with Stage 3 breast cancer.

When Sue told me she had breast cancer, I, like many she told, was stunned. I started to cry. She said firmly, "No tears. I need only positivity." She had recently lost a job she loved, and it seemed unfairly cruel. Again. "Nope...it's their loss, I know there's something better for me around the corner." As promised, I didn't cry in front of her and remained as optimistic and positive as possible.

At the time, my husband and I were planning our annual Survivor Crop Fundraising event, a 24-hour crafting marathon that brought passionate people together to raise funds and awareness for breast cancer. That year, we asked her to volunteer with planning the event and she gladly hit the ground running.

Somedays it was surreal. Actually, nearly every memory I have of Sue's experience fighting "The BC Beast" was unreal. Over the course of roughly two years, her positive attitude and creative spirit were infectious. She left no wiggle room for the rest of us to "feel sorry" for her. She was fighting the battle of her life and she was going to fight hard. I remember her making us laugh when she donned her bodacious bald head in her leather biker vest.

Sue would bring a sprinkle of creative dust to the Chemo Center. She would leave a trail of joy that was certainly not there before she walked in the doors. She and her sister would bring chemo crafting kits so she'd have something positive and fun to focus on while she was receiving her infusions.

Even on Sue's worst days (I remember the heat radiating from her scorched skin), she was determined to beat cancer. And she did. While working full time during the Great Recession. Moment by Moment. Day by Day. Every harrowing step of her journey she faced with bravery, uncommon wit, humor, and sass. This is her story of how she "survived" the shipwreck and got off that island. I pray that her story will give hope and strength to all who read it.

—Camille Akin

Friend, Fellow Crafter, Passionate about Helping Women

Words That Gave Me Strength

Cancer is a word, not a sentence.

— John Diamond

Attitudes are contagious. Are yours worth catching?

— Dennis and Wendy Mannering

Write it on your heart that every day is the best day in the year.

— Ralph Waldo Emerson

Courage is not the absence of fear, but rather the judgment that something else is more important than fear.

— Ambrose Redmoon

The person who can bring the spirit of laughter into a room is indeed blessed.

— Bennett Cerf

Optimism is the foundation of courage.

— Nicholas Murray Butler

Courage is being scared to death, but saddling up anyway.

– John Wayne

Life Happens

Celebrating a wonderful 30-year career anniversary followed by life changing events was not in my plan. But then again, you can't deal your cards and play them too.

It was fall, 2007. Times were changing. The financial Armageddon was lurking around the corner. The housing market was about to crash. 2.6 million hardworking people were losing their jobs, the worst in 60 years. It was the beginning of the Great Recession. There was no discrimination. Loyalty was lost. We were warned at work that layoffs were coming and my colleagues and I were collectively worried about the impending doom.

In spring of 2008, in preparation for possibly losing my health benefits, I scheduled a physical and mammogram. The mammogram showed two pinhead calcifications on one breast. I was re-scheduled for another mammogram three days later. The secondary results indicated nothing serious, but I would have a follow-up exam in six months.

After 30 incredible years with Hewlett-Packard, (HP) a company that I loved, respected, and whose products I proudly evangelized, my new boss of three months simply read me a form letter stating that I was one of 45% of the marketing department layoff. Sorry it didn't work out. That was in April, but my termination date wasn't until August.

I slowly plodded back to my desk with the embarrassing manila envelope in my hand. I started packing up my office. As I glanced up and down the hallways, I spied a couple of other colleagues with glum faces, and their own manilla envelope bearing the news. I won't pretend it didn't hurt. I felt like my spouse of 30 years had cheated on me. Until this moment, I had never had a devastating loss. This simply was the most negative thing that had rocked my world. I stewed for a couple of months, then decided to get over it and return to my typically cheerful self.

It was really important to me to work for another company that made cool products, and Sony was on the top of my list. We've always owned Sony TVs, a Walkman in the 80s, and a Handycam when our first son was born. Plus, it was directly across the street from where I had worked for the past 30 years. My car knew the route and could simply make a right turn instead of a left to get to the office.

I applied for a marketing job in September that was a perfect match with my talent and expertise. I really hoped to land an interview.

I scheduled the six-month follow up mammogram for the end of September. I had the mammogram, and three days later my doctor called to say that I needed to have a biopsy on two suspicious calcifications. The biopsy was scheduled for the following Monday, October 6.

The next day, I received a call from the clinic, to make an appointment with a surgical nurse. Being confused, I thought she was referring to the biopsy, and I told her that I already had my biopsy scheduled for Monday. She continued by saying that my appointment would be on Tuesday, October 14th. I was clueless as to what the appointment was for, and figured it was simply a follow-up.

Shortly after that call, I was thrilled when Sony called asking me to come in for an interview...on Monday. I of course agreed to the much-needed interview, then called the scheduler to change my biopsy appointment. Let me tell you, the scheduler was not happy that I moved the biopsy, but I explained that I was unemployed and desperately needed a job.

I knew that delaying the biopsy by 24 hours was not going to kill me.

Monday morning, I went to the interview and was greeted with a panel of three managers. I've always enjoyed panel interviews as everyone gets to hear all the questions and answers, with no room for misinterpretation. The interview went well and I was confident that I nailed it. The Marketing Director asked me the tough question, "How did you feel about being laid off after 30 years?" I honestly told her that it was tough at first, but I was one of 45% of the marketing department that got laid off. I couldn't take that personally. Plus, I had 30 incredible years there and multitudes of friends that I kept in contact with via Facebook and the Retiree's Club. Now I simply had to wait patiently for a job offer.

The day after my interview I went in for the biopsy, not realizing what an adventure it would be. Women over 40 all know the experience of having their breasts placed in a vice grip that cranks tighter and tighter, "just a little bit more." Good grief, I had no idea that for the biopsy, you not only get squashed tighter, but you also have to remain in that way more than uncomfortable position for about 45 minutes.

The procedure began by locating one spot with computerized equipment, and then numbing me with a burning injection. The nurse's claim that it just burns a little was unfounded. It hurt like hell. She then made an incision followed by suctioning out the suspicious cells, then took them to the lab to determine if they were cancerous. She finally released the grip, and I turned over so she could put pressure on the incision, and placed a steri-strip to close it.

Breathe in, breathe out. Keep breathing. This, too shall pass.

Five minutes later, I turned over to start the same grueling procedure on the second spot. Thank god the second one was much easier and only took about 20 minutes. For those of you of the male gender reading this, who can't imagine what it feels like, just replace the word breast with your favorite private part. Then you'll get it.

The three nurses who worked on the biopsies were very kind and informative, which I like. I don't like surprises. Before I left, they gave me "A Woman's Guide to Breast

Cancer Diagnosis and Treatment." They told me not to read it, as it would probably scare me.

"Eighty-five percent of the women who have biopsies don't have cancer, so there's no use in getting worked up over it if no cancer is found," she explained. I liked her logic and tossed the booklet on the nightstand when I got home.

My primary doctor would receive the results Thursday or Friday, and he would call me with the update. Thursday and Friday came, and I didn't receive a call. I called my doctor's office on Friday afternoon and was told that he was out and wouldn't be in until Monday. I asked if anyone else could give me the results and was told no. I was assured he would call on Monday.

In this age of technology, it's very easy to do your own homework. Being frustrated and kept in the dark as to why I was having an appointment on Tuesday, I Googled the nurse's name and clinic and discovered that she was a surgical nurse in the breast cancer care center. She was listed along with other oncologists, radiologists, and plastic surgeons.

Bingo! I definitely had cancer, but still had not been officially informed.

I told nobody. There was no reason to freak anyone out when I simply did not have enough information yet. I pushed cancer out of my mind and carried on with my weekend. I'm not one to fabricate what-if scenarios. Once I had the medical facts, I would start my plan of attack.

Monday morning my doctor finally called. This is verbatim. "Hello, Susan? I'm calling to see if you've made an appointment with the surgeon yet." He didn't identify himself, but I recognized his trembling voice.

"Yes, I have an appointment with a surgical nurse in the morning."

"Good, good, because your results came back and you have cancer."

"Yes," I sarcastically snapped, "I already discovered online that she's a breast cancer surgical nurse." I mentally slammed down the phone, then changed to a different general practitioner. To say he was bedside manner challenged was putting it mildly.

It was crucial that I had open and honest communication with my team of doctors. I needed to trust and believe in them. My former doctor knew for two weeks that I had two tumors, which was validated with the biopsy. Yet, he couldn't bear to deliver the news until the last minute.

My volcano was about to erupt!

The Spiel

I literally shed two tears and decided right then and there, this was not a crying matter. I needed to beat it, and that wasn't going to work with a pathetic, feel-sorry-for-myself-attitude. I had to focus all my energy on beating cancer, not on asking why me. It is what it is and plenty of people have been diagnosed with and beaten cancer. I would be one of the winners.

I summoned up my Mary Poppins attitude, put on a happy face and quickly put together my spiel. I needed to nail it so that I could convincingly deliver the message to family and friends. I knew that if I was upbeat and fighting to win, my attitude would be contagious. Friends and family would be moved to join me in the positive fight, rather than mourn the bump in the road.

I knew it would be easier over the phone. At least if they started crying silent tears, I wouldn't have to see them. I couldn't be sucked into their tornado of feelings, spinning out of control.

It's not fair! Why you? You've lost your job, now you have cancer. Oh my god you have to do chemo! Your hair will fall out! Yadda, yadda, yadda.

The first call was to my best friend. I knew she would be the perfect person to test drive my spiel. I wanted to have it rock solid before breaking the news to my family.

"Hi, it's me. I'm going to be okay, I'm going to be fine, but I've been diagnosed with breast cancer. I'm going to kick it in the ass with a positive and upbeat attitude. If you have the need to cry or have a meltdown, you need to do it on your own time, away from me and the phone."

Pamela was very calm and collected. I told her I would go to the doctor the next day and find out just how extensive it was and what the treatment plan would be to ensure that I obliterated it from my body.

After about three minutes of conversation, she abruptly said, "I gotta go, I'll call you back." This wasn't unusual for Pamela, and I figured that her dog Dottie had just pooped on the floor again. It was a daily routine and I knew it well.

As she explained a few hours later when she called me back, she was starting to lose it, and knew I didn't want to hear it. She sobbed for a short while, and then decided she had to get over it and be supportive for my sake. She was scared. Really scared. But this wasn't about her. She knew that I would need all my energy fixated on slaying the beast. I couldn't use one iota of inner strength to comfort distraught, fearful friends.

I felt empowered. My spiel worked on my first friend. On to the next. I called her and delivered the spiel. She, too, handled it very well and even joked about if I had to have a mastectomy, she'd get a boob job with me when the time was right for reconstruction. Friends definitely handled it well.

I knew that Denny, my sweet, sentimental husband would not fare as well. Neither would my sister Sandra, who lost her husband to colon cancer 16 years prior. She would still tear up at the sight of an X-ray, because Jim's final X-ray revealed that cancer had taken over his liver, lungs, and the rest of his colon. Not long after his terminal diagnosis, hospice was brought into their home to help with his comfort and care during his transition. He lost his brief battle just four days after their first anniversary.

Denny came home a little while later and asked, "Did you hear from the doctor?" I quickly launched into my spiel. I was very proud of him as he didn't fall apart as he normally would have. He was so brave around me and only had his moments of crying with other relatives and friends.

"I have to do this positively. I can't wear myself down with sadness and crying. It just won't work." He was scared. He feared he'd lose me. I wasn't afraid. I knew I could beat it. I was determined to focus on the challenge. I would claim victory with an Oscar-worthy upbeat performance.

Next, I called Sandra at work. I didn't want to tell her over the phone, but I also didn't want her to hear it from anyone else. Plus, I knew she'd lose it if I told her in person. Her knees buckled as she gripped the phone. Her voice cracked a couple of times, but she held it together for my sake. Six hours later, she came traipsing through the back door. She took one look at me and asked "Did we really have that conversation this morning? Is it true?" She desperately wanted to believe it was a bad dream.

"Yes, we did. It wasn't a dream. According to statistics, one in eight women get breast cancer. I took the hit for our family, so you're good to go," I said with a grin.

She high-fived me and enthusiastically said, "Thanks, Sis!" I reassured her that I was fighting to win. I would kill cancer. It wouldn't kill me. This was breast cancer, and we caught it early. I would slay the beast and she would play a crucial, creative role, in helping me fight the battle with a happy face. She just didn't know it yet.

Plan B

Tuesday morning was a sunny SoCal day. There was a thickness in the air as Denny and I prepared to meet the challenge, find out just what state my body was in, and to determine the plan of attack. We headed out to our favorite breakfast spot Champagne French Bakery in Carmel Mountain, and chit-chatted about our boys. We avoided the C-word, because we just didn't have enough information yet. No sense worrying about what might be. We would know in a few short hours how to gear up, face the enemy, and kick it in the royal ass.

As we sat in the surgeon's waiting room, there was a very sad, depressed 20-something year old woman, who was clearly a cancer patient. She was dressed like a drab nun wearing a black skirt, grey blouse, and a black scarf to hide her bald head. She was not handling cancer well and her eyes were red and swollen from crying. She plodded into the office as though heading to the guillotine.

That's not me. I won't do depression. I won't wear a scarf. I won't cry. I will laugh all the way to victory. I will kill cancer. It won't get the best of me. I am a winner! Look out cancer – here I come.

The time arrived and we were called in to greet the challenge. I really liked the Nurse Who Must Not Be Named – at first. She had yet to reveal her true colors, and I'm not talking about yellow beams of sunshine and daffodils of joy. She was very matter of fact, and told me that I had two tumors, on opposite sides of my left breast. One was HER2-positive and the other was DCIS. DCIS is a very early form of cancer that is noninvasive, while HER2 positive is very invasive.

I would have a mastectomy, six months of chemo, and at least six weeks of radiation. She said we wouldn't know the stage of the cancer until surgery, because the stage is determined by how far cancer has spread, and if it was invading other organs or lymph nodes. So now we knew. It was bad, but maybe not that bad. Women are cured of breast cancer all the time. Sure, there are those who don't make it, but there are many who do.

I'm going to be one of those winners. I will fight the fight. I will never give up. It's just a body part. Hell, it's done its part and fed our babies. It's really quite useless, except for making me look like a balanced woman, rather than the Cyclops I was about to become. Whatever. Charge on to battle and don't hesitate.

I was psyched. It was my real life video game challenge, and the enemy would go down in flames, or at least in a chemo cocktail or two.

The surgeon, Dr. Kurtzhals, came in next, and I immediately fell in love with her. She was young, upbeat, and reiterated how we were going to eliminate the snarling beast invading my body. She showed me photos of women before and after surgery, along with the miraculous final photos post reconstruction. We chose a plastic surgeon, who down the road would magically re-build a new perky breast, to replace the lemon that had sprouted from my chest. Like many other strong women before me, I decided to make refreshing pink lemonade from the lemon I was given. Just add a dose of sweet friends, warm hugs, and many shots of laughter.

After thoroughly explaining the extensive list of upcoming medical procedures from mastectomy, to chemo, to radiation, and finally reconstruction, the doctor routinely inquired "Do you have any questions for me?"

"Yes, how soon after the mastectomy can I go back to work?"

She laughed and said "With your attitude, five to seven days. The poor woman who just left my office was sobbing and wanted 20-22 weeks off from work. She's going to have a very long road ahead of her."

"Great, because I had an interview a week ago and I feel very confident about it. If they offer me the job, I want to start working as soon as possible."

Yes, I will kick it with my attitude. I can do this!

She assured me that my approach would guarantee a technical knockout with several rounds of chemo cocktails and a few weeks at "the tanning salon," my pet name for the radiation lab. For me, joking about the countless number of treatments, kept my spirits up. My laughter put people at ease, and put their tears at bay...most of the time.

Thus, began my journey down the winding, bumpy path to cancer FREEdom. Bound and determined to keep the upbeat attitude, I forged ahead planning for the upcoming surgery and treatment. When the scheduler called to say my surgery would be November 4th at 7:00 a.m., I emphatically asked if I could move it later in the day. Surprised, she said, "yes," and reiterated that I couldn't eat until after the surgery.

"Yes, I know, but its Election Day and I want to vote." There was no sense letting a little surgery get in the way of my civic duties. This was just another step in proving that cancer was not controlling me and taking charge of my life. I might have to bend to the ways of the cocktails and spa treatments, but I was going to call the shots whenever possible.

I was most excited to meet the plastic surgeon to see how she would work her magic for reconstruction. Dr. Arya gave us the low down on what was ahead, once we cleared the chemo and radiation paths. She was another empathetic and artistic doctor who was very friendly, open, and explained everything in great detail. She did not recommend immediate reconstruction, as the implant expander, which is slowly filled with saline to stretch the skin in preparation for the real implant, tends to get in the way of the radiation treatment. After the mastectomy healed, I would have a prosthesis to wear to even me out until the time was right for reconstruction.

She explained in detail that there were two different options available for reconstruction. The first was a tram flap where skin and fat is taken from the abdomen. Can you say tummy tuck? The second option was a latissimus dorsi flap, where skin and muscle are harvested from the back and grafted onto the chest. Since I didn't have enough "extra" in my stomach, which is probably a good thing, she would take the skin graft and other tissues from my back.

The procedure would involve making an incision just under the left shoulder blade to cut out a football shaped piece of skin, a slice of the latissimus muscle, fat, and blood vessels. They would be moved to my chest to reconstruct the breast and help support the implant. I had two very good friends, plus my sister, who offered to be tummy tuck donors, but the surgeon insisted that she would have to use my parts.

I was so sorry to disappoint the would-be donors, but damn, I had my own replacement parts ready and waiting. Let's do this.

I was getting anxious about the mastectomy and trying to prepare for the next few months with drastic bodily changes. I was planning what type of wardrobe I would create to disguise my misshapen body. I figured open vests, with a soft button up shirt underneath, would be a great solution. I wanted to be able to get dressed easily with minimal chest and arm movements, so front opening tops would be key. The open vests would serve to stand out in the front and create the illusion that I had twin peaks, and not a peak with a nearby mesa. Surely the illusion of my chest was insignificant compared to the possible inconvenience of being dead.

My next appointment prior to the mastectomy was for an MRI. The doctor wanted to get another look at the tumors, prior to surgery. I knew about the part where they put you into this long space ship looking machine, but actually doing it was pretty weird and extremely claustrophobic. The head phones and country music really helped keep me calm, but damn, did that machine make some loud-ass noises.

The noises were all a bit different, from whirring and humming to a noise similar to a Lear jet taking off. But the lovely lady behind the curtain would interrupt every so often and quietly tell me which new sound I would hear and how long it would last, so I wouldn't be startled. Overall, it wasn't too bad, but then I had taken some kind of loopy drug just prior, so I really couldn't care less about what was happening.

My radiation oncologist, Dr. Lin, was the third doctor to join our team of experts, and we really liked him too. Not only was he knowledgeable, compassionate, and very thorough in his explanation of treatment, he also was a hugger, which I love.

He showed us the MRI, which was a very clear picture of how large the tumors were. The one spot was less than

1/4 inch, but the second one was even larger. It was very scary that the tumors could grow that fast in only six months. There also was a new small spot on the right breast, so I would soon be going in for another mammogram and ultrasound. Advertisement: Ladies, and guys start nagging your ladies, go get that mammogram – it could save your/her life.

Dr. Lin told us that I would most likely have chemo for four months, followed by seven weeks of radiation, because the cancer was so invasive. We were hoping the price of gas would go down because my SUV gas sucking hog would be hauling my butt 35 miles to San Diego five days a week for seven weeks.

I felt it was critical to get a second opinion. Not that I didn't trust my doctors, but this was a huge medical ordeal that was going to wreak havoc on my body. I wanted to be double sure that the plan of attack was going to be successful. I wanted a professional opinion from a doctor outside of my network. Plus, each one of my doctors encouraged me to get a second opinion, to ensure the treatment plan was spot on.

My brother, Scott, is one of the most well-connected people I know. He told his best friend, about my diagnosis, and Bim told him that he has a cousin who is a very prominent breast surgeon in New York. Within 10 minutes, I was on the phone with Dr. Alison Estabrook, Chief of the Comprehensive Breast Center, Mount Sinai-Roosevelt Hospital in New York City. She was such a sweet, warm, and caring person. I explained my situation to her and she asked me to fax my mammogram and pathology reports to her so she could look at them. She agreed with the course of treatment that my doctors had recommended. I was so relieved to hear from another expert professional that I was on the right path to success.

She then called a friend, a breast surgeon in San Diego, to see if she could see me. Dr. Julie Barone, left me a voicemail about 20 minutes later saying that I could call her assistant in the morning and ask her to fit me in that day. And she did! Wow – talk about connections.

Big thanks to my favorite bro. When thrown the cancer curve ball I talked about my diagnosis and possible treatment with close friends and family. It was important to take advantage of any connections that they might have in the medical field, because I trusted that they were looking out for my best interest.

I called Dr. Barone's office first thing in the morning, and got an appointment with her at 3:00 the same day. It was unbelievably cool that she took me in with practically no notice. She too was very professional and informative. We talked in her office for nearly an hour, and then she examined me.

The only thing she differed on is that she would recommend doing the expansion implant right away and the full re-construction later. But, she did not have the advantage of seeing the MRI and mammogram, because she was in an entirely different hospital network. It was reassuring to hear from yet another doctor that my doctors in my medical group were on the right path to wiping out the cancer invading my body.

There are usually three huge fears when diagnosed with cancer — death, vomiting uncontrollably, and hair loss. I had already decided that my Mary Poppins attitude would fend off death and vomiting, but I couldn't stop the hair loss. I decided to make the best of it. I bought an incredible wig that looked just like my hair, and then decided that I would have fun yanking it off to freak out unsuspecting people.

My friend Lillian, who had been recently diagnosed with breast cancer, was going through chemo, and had the most incredible wig that looked exactly like her real hair. She took me to see Patti Joyce, a delightful two-time cancer survivor, who designs and styles wigs in her home boutique in Carlsbad. www.wigsbypattispearls.com

Patti retired from Hollywood where she used to make wigs for movie and TV stars. She then dedicated her life to helping women overcome their fear of losing their hair to chemo, by helping them choose a wig that would make them feel beautiful.

The first wig I tried on was too blonde, too long in the front, and hung down around my chin. It felt like a spider crawling on my neck and gave me the heebie-jeebies. I tried on a couple more, and finally, found the one that was just right. I loved it. The color was exactly like mine, dark with blonde highlights, and the cut was similar to my own hair.

It was a bit too thick, but she would thin it out for me and style it prior to my going bald. I was super excited to be able to instantly replace my hair when it started falling out.

November 4th was a drizzly day, but it didn't dampen my spirits. Denny and I were first in line at the polls to cast our votes. Because it was raining, traffic was a nightmare. Since we southern Californians get so little rain, it wreaks havoc on traffic. The oils that have dripped from vehicles rise to the surface and endless accidents ensue. Lord knows, you can't slow down and drive like a cautious and responsible driver, because getting to work on time is so critically important to your welfare.

We slowly cruised down highways 15, 56, and 5 to the hospital overlooking the beautiful Pacific Ocean. We were 45 minutes late for our appointment, but so was everyone else, doctors, nurses, and patients included. I was anxious to have the pesky lemon plucked from my chest and thrown into the bad apple bin.

Get this sucker off my chest!

One of the preparations for surgery was to inject me with a radioactive dye, one hour before the surgery. The dye would go through my lymphatic system and would indicate whether or not the cancer had spread to my lymph nodes. I'm not a fan of needles, and was quite nervous about the one that they'd insert into my nipple. Yep by golly, it hurt all right, but it wasn't as excruciating as another one coming around the bend. More on that later.

The surgery went well and took about two and a half hours, but they also discovered that the cancer had spread to 11 lymph nodes, thereby resulting in a Stage three diagnosis. Stage four, the worst, is having it metastasize into major nearby organs, and thankfully that didn't happen because we caught it early.

The process for testing lymph nodes is very methodical. Because lymph nodes are attached linearly, similar to old school Christmas lights where you pull out a light and replace it with a new one to see if it was the bad one, they removed the first two nodes and checked for cancer. The nodes tested positive, so they took two more. This continued until they found a clean lymph node. Lymph node number 12 was clean as a whistle, so they were done.

After surgery, the doctor came out to talk with my worried husband and sister. She kneeled down in front of Denny and put her hands on his knees. Denny immediately jumped to conclusions that something went horribly wrong and he panicked. She was simply being thoughtful and caring, looked him in the eyes, and said the surgery was successful and I would be fine. I spent the night in the hospital and was released the next day. It really wasn't that big of deal and wasn't nearly as painful as the bunion surgery I had earlier in the year. Sure, I was sore, and couldn't move my left arm much, but heck, that's why I was given a prescription for oxycodone.

One thing that was really annoying was the JP drain protruding from my back. It made sleeping feel like a bad camping trip where as many times as you try to adjust to get comfortable, you still have that gnarly tree root poking you in the back. I kept reminding myself that it was only temporary, and the drain would be removed in a week or so.

Breathe. Stay positive. Keep laughing. I can do this.

I prayed a silent prayer of thanks. I was thrilled that the cancer was found early, and it had only spread to a few lymph nodes. I indulged in reading numerous books to take my mind off the distraction of cancer. One of my favorites was *Three Cups of Tea* by Greg Mortenson. It's a very inspirational story about one man's quest to make a difference in the lives of children in Pakistan and Afghanistan, by building schools for them. I read many books during my recuperation, and selected mostly uplifting ones, to keep me focused on positivity.

The week after my mastectomy, I went for a scheduled visit to have the JP drain removed from my back. I brought with me my obligatory chart showing how many cc of fluid was emptied several times each day. When it got down to less than 30cc accumulated in a 24-hour period, the drain could be removed. The fluid level was down, but that was due to the drain line being partially clogged.

This was where the Nurse Who Must Not Be Named earned her new name, Nurse Ratched. Her true evil colors began to shine. She kicked off my visit by snapping at me and demanded to know why I hadn't been milking the drain line to clean it. Shocked at her attitude, I told her that

I wasn't aware that I had to milk the line, as it wasn't listed in my post-op procedures.

Milking consisted of squeezing the line tightly then sliding her fingers down the line to force the clogged fluid into the drain bulb. She started the procedure and each and every effing time she released the line before compressing and milking again. The line created a vacuum and excruciatingly sucked fluid out of my back. It felt like a dagger was being plunged into me with each milking.

I kept biting my tongue as a distraction, and had tears rolling down my face as she did this a dozen or more times. Denny was horrified that I was in so much pain. When she finished, she glared at Denny and barked, "You're going to have to do this for her at home!"

"I can't do that. I can't hurt her," he quietly muttered.

Clearly since Denny wasn't going to help, I would have to do it myself. I knew I would figure out how to milk the line pain-free, and I did. The trick was to never release the line until the very end. Yes, my fingers were cramping from squeezing the line for so long, but as soon as I reached the end of the line, I very slowly released the pressure on the line. Voila! No pain at all from milking.

When I went back for the next visit, I saw another nurse, and I made sure to educate her about the proper way of milking a line. She thanked me for the tip and added that Nurse Ratched must have forgotten to open the air release on the bulb, which caused the vacuum. I seriously wondered how many others she had tortured over the years. She was truly the most insensitive and cruel nurse that I've ever encountered.

Cocktails Anyone?

We met with my chemo oncologist several days after the milking debacle. We called her the bartender because she would create designer cocktails just for me. Wasn't that special?

Dr. Kroener, another warm, caring, and extraordinary professional, was concerned that the cancer had spread into 11 lymph nodes and said they'd have to be more aggressive with the chemo. We would start with one cocktail of Adriamycin, Cytoxan, Benadryl, and Emend, every three weeks for 12 weeks, followed by another recipe of Taxol, Herceptin, Benadryl, and Emend, for 12 more weekly infusions. She gave me a cryptic note with abbreviated names on them, but I was almost certain they would not be as yummy as a mojito or a strawberry daiquiri.

The first chemo infusion was scheduled for the day before Thanksgiving. Since Thanksgiving has always been my favorite meal to cook, I planned to prepare the fresh pumpkin two days early, in case I wasn't feeling well on Wednesday evening. I figured this would also be a great opportunity to give the boys a crash course in cooking turkey, stuffing, pumpkin pie, and appetizers.

In preparation for chemo, there was an onslaught of tests that had to be done. I was seriously starting to feel like a pin cushion. Countless needles, scans, echocardiograms, and MRIs. First up was the echocardiogram. The technician used a transducer with gel on it to glide over my chest, sending ultrasonic sound waves that bounce back to create images of the heart. These echoes are sent to a computer, which creates moving photos of the valves and chambers. These records were kept in my file for comparison, to see if the chemo does any damage to my heart in the future.

It all was going well, until the tech got to a certain part that was obscured by scar tissue from my mastectomy. Try as he might, he just couldn't get a good picture. He tried applying more pressure, which was very painful. Trying to make light of the moment, I was thinking to myself, how could scar tissue obstruct the view when there wasn't even a breast in the way?

The only solution was to give me an IV with a contrast so they could see what's happening in the area. The trouble was the nurse tried four times and couldn't get a good stick. She finally called in the reinforcements.

The new nurse wrapped my arm with a tourniquet, had me hang it down by my side for three minutes, and then was able to get a good stick the first time. I asked if they could leave in the catheter for my 11:30 appointment, because I would need another contrast for the PET scan.

The nurse called in the cardiologist and he said while they're really not supposed to let a patient leave with it in, he didn't think I looked like a child of the 60s who would relish the opportunity to have a clear avenue for recreational drugs. Woo-hoo, I didn't need to have yet another nurse struggle with finding a vein. Another simple thankful moment.

When I arrived at the clinic, the techs and nurses there were surprised, but pleased that I already had a catheter in place due to my bad sticks at the other office.

I was met with a delay due to scanner malfunctions. Having worked for a technology company for 30 years, I was more than used to technical glitches when equipment failed to cooperate.

Being the prepared person that I was, I blissfully sat and read Lance Armstrong's book, It's *Not About the Bike*, while waiting for the equipment to be repaired. My brother Jerry, thoughtfully sent me this book when I was diagnosed with cancer. I found this book very inspirational as Lance used his kick-butt attitude to help fight his own brain cancer battle.

I found many of these procedures both fascinating and interesting. Thanks to the Internet, it was so easy to study the procedures and side effects prior to the appointment. This helped make the process logical and less emotional.

The next test was a combination of a computed tomography (CT) scan and a positron emission tomography (PET) scan. The CT scan showed details of internal organs, and the PET scan showed malignant versus benign cells. It involved injecting a radioactive chemical, which is absorbed into the cells, providing better visibility. I laid down on the imaging table, which moves inside the scanner as it takes a CT digital x-ray to create a topogram. Then the PET scan was conducted to locate the malignant cells. The whole process from injection to scan took nearly two hours.

After that, I just headed back home to the hum drum normalcy of my life in beautiful sunny SoCal. Much to my surprise, when I arrived home there was beautiful flower arrangement greeting me from my friends John and Jeanne deMeules. I'm telling you, there is nothing better than HP friends who stick by you to the end. It meant so much to me that they sent the beautiful gesture of hope and positive vibes to keep me kicking cancer in the ass.

The following week I had three HP co-workers who came to visit. Liz Phillips, my sweet friend from marketing came by for a short visit. She also brought our family a scrumptious lasagna dinner, complete with salad and garlic bread.

The next two visitors who came were friends who I met during my time in accounting. Kasey Mayfield, my hilarious friend who kept the whole office laughing, and the talented Bobbie Zinker, who is one of the best quilters that I've ever known.

Bobbie made a gorgeous handmade quilt for a breast cancer fundraiser, at the request of a friend. The quilt was put into a silent auction, with no opening bid. At the end of the evening, the highest bid was $100, so the friend who donated it upped the bid to $110 and won the quilt. She then gave the quilt back to Bobbie.

Bobbie said she'd give to the next woman diagnosed with breast cancer, and I was the lucky winner! See how easy it is to be upbeat and positive when you have friends who give you a priceless gift? The gorgeous handmade quilt decorates my home with love, thoughtfulness, and warm memories of my sweet friend.

This piece of art is my favorite conversation starter in my home. I too am a quilter, but I've never made a quilt that is this magnificent. Bobbie, hand-stitched all the vines and flowers onto the quilt squares, then stitched all the blocks together to make the finished quilt.

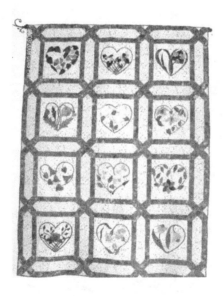

Handmade quilt from Bobbie Zinker

Two weeks after my surgery, my neighbor, Karen Garcia, and I went to go pick up my wig. She was so cute when I told her I wanted to go get it that week, before I started chemo. I told her I had a couple of girlfriends that offered to go with me, but she insisted, "No, please call me first."

She drove us over to Patti's boutique in Carlsbad. As I sat in the vanity chair and Patti was putting on and adjusting my wig, Karen just sat there and stared at me in awe. She couldn't believe how real the wig looked. Patti trimmed it a bit more for me, and just as we were getting ready to leave, another couple arrived for their appointment.

They were a husband and wife in their 70s, and the woman was undergoing treatment for colon cancer. The man looked at Karen and me and said, "You ladies don't look like you belong here."

I piped up with, "One of us does."

"Who?"

"It's me. I came and picked out my wig before losing my hair, so I could be sure it would look just like my real hair. What do you think?"

He stared in disbelief. His wife had a really awful looking wig, similar to the one Julia Roberts wore in Mother's Day. She was there to get a new one that not only looked real, but would also make her feel beautiful. They were astonished that I was wearing a wig and kept remarking at how natural it looked. His wife's mood changed, and she transformed from looking sad and depressed, to being excited about the possibility of a natural and realistic looking wig.

We headed over to Pelly's, the amazing fish taco restaurant, and ordered lunch. We sat and chatted, and she just kept staring at me and my wig. We made the scenic drive home along Del Dios Highway and took in the sights of the hillsides and Lake Hodges dam.

I was anxious to get to Karen's house so that I could ask her husband, Mike, an ER doctor, his opinion about getting a port for chemo, rather than having an IV inserted for each treatment. Mike highly recommended a port for two reasons. First, only my right arm could be used for an IV because the removal of lymph nodes from my left prevented me from ever having needle sticks in my left arm again. Second, because my right arm would be used for all the IVs for blood draws, chemo, and contrasts for scans, my veins would be prone to collapsing from being over used. I would most-likely develop scar tissue from the numerous sticks which could also impede easy sticks in the future.

Karen and I wanted to see if he noticed it was a wig. He definitely did because he kept shifting his eyes from my wig to my eyes, but he politely didn't say anything to me.

From there I went to pick up my 16 year old son, Kyle from school and took him to get his driver's license. He passed with flying colors and was so excited that he never even noticed that I was wearing a wig.

After that, we stopped by Burger King to feed the starving teen. Sean, the boys' best friend who was living with us, was working the drive-through. He too had no clue that I was wearing a wig. Okay, they're teenage boys and didn't notice too much about women, unless they were teenagers.

Ka-ching! I had faked out four out of six people so far.

When I got home, Tyler, my 19-year-old was there, and I could tell immediately that he knew it was a wig, because he kept looking at my hair. But, being the polite and courteous teen that he was, he never said a word.

The best part was when Denny came home a while later. We had dinner and sat at the dining room table chatting for at least 40 minutes before he said, "Hey, did you and Karen make it over to the wig place today?"

I was amused and just smirked at him.

"No, you're not wearing it are you? How can I have known you for 24 years and not recognized that that was not your real hair?"

Pretty. Freaking. Funny.

As you can imagine, my fear of going bald had now totally diminished. Who cares? I could immediately pop on my wig and have insta-hair. Plus, my friend, Donna Johnson, told me she knew how to put on fake eyelashes – too cool. My newly purchased incognito accessory would assist me in my quest for continuing my upbeat kick-cancer-in-the-ass attitude.

The next couple of weeks were uneventful, and I spent my time reading, sewing, and regaining my strength. When I finally had the drain removed, I became much more mobile and loved getting back to exercising and walking. I had purchased the Wii Fit gaming system for my sons the prior year, but they thought it was hokey. I tried it for myself and loved it. I especially liked the steps, yoga, skiing, boxing and jogging.

What I found interesting was that I actually scored better in yoga and the balance games post-surgery. Because I couldn't raise my left arm above my shoulder, it helped me to have better balance. I felt like I was cheating, but I really didn't have a choice as my mobility with my arm was very compromised. I was able to unlock the advanced step, and some longer repetitions with lunges, and with the more challenging exercises I gained much more strength.

I also started my walking routine again, which was so invigorating. I lived in a beautiful neighborhood of Hidden Meadows. There were many challenging hills to climb and a variety of organic ranches along the way. The hills were decorated with macadamia groves, vineyards, kiwi farms, and many citrus groves of blood oranges, tangerines, oranges, lemons, limes, and grapefruit. Plus, the friendly horses down the road loved the apple and carrot snacks that I would bring them for a treat. You just can't beat the sunshine, fresh air, and beautiful landscapes in southern

California. It only took me a few short weeks to return to my typical four-mile walking routine.

Working for a Living

A week after my mastectomy, I finally got the call I was hoping for from Sony, and would be going back to work the week of Thanksgiving. I was hired as a contract marketer, and it was so exciting to be working again and for a cool electronics firm. I kept pushing my exercise routine, to help build up my strength before starting full-time work along with the chemo routine.

I took advantage of my last two weeks of unemployment to finish up making handmade Christmas cards, handmade ornaments for friends, as well as finishing a couple of quilted wall hangings.

One afternoon, just before going back to work, I was going through all my cancer literature and came across the instructions for physical therapy. Because I had 12 lymph nodes removed from my armpit and arm, I developed cording, which is a cord-like band under my arm. It compromised my mobility and I couldn't stretch my arm any further than 90 degrees from my side. The goal was to be able to move my arm vertically, so that it would be straight up at 180 degrees, just as it was prior to surgery.

I had remembered what the physical therapist told me in the hospital, and to be honest with you, I was doing some exercises, but clearly not as much as I was supposed to do.

So, I dug right in and started the stretches and movement that would expedite rejuvenating my flexibility.

I did the second round of stretches in my kitchen facing the wall of measurements. This wall has all the growth charts for my kids and grandkids, and even the dreaded beer belly measurements of my three brothers. The last time we were all together, was for my 50th birthday bash. OMG, it was so freaking funny to see my never-had-a-beer-gut-in-his-life middle brother next to the other two. I'll leave it at that.

My exercise consisted of standing six inches away from the wall, and reaching up with my right (good) hand as far as I could, and marking the spot with tape. Then, I had to do my let-your-fingers-do-the-walking exercise to inch my left hand up the wall to try to get it as far as the right hand could reach. As I was doing this, I was carrying on a conversation with my six-foot one-inch son, Kyle. After the third reaching exercise he asked me what I was doing. I told him I was working on trying to reach the tape I put on the wall with my right hand. Without skipping a beat, he asked, "Why didn't you just ask me to do it?"

The fact that he was clueless as to the point of the exercise really hit a chord with me and I busted up laughing. OK, humor me, I was looking for entertainment. One more day until I'd be back into the throes of employment. I was super excited, and hoped that they would "get it" that I really was going to kick-ass and do a great job – in spite of chemo and radiation treatments.

Now came the tough part, formulating a plan to break the news to my new employer. I knew I would be every employer's worst nightmare, starting a job with a life-threatening disease. But it wasn't really threatening my life, because I was going to beat it! I just had to convince them that I could make it real.

I'm a very honest person and not very good at lying. I was worried about not being upfront with my employer when they hired me. I called a good friend of mine, a manager at HP, to get her advice on when to tell them about my health. I gave Veneeta Eason the spiel, and she took it extremely well. Her voice never cracked, and she told me very professionally that I didn't have to tell them anything until it was time to miss work for treatments. I decided I'd tell my new boss right before my first chemo.

What I didn't know, and I found out a couple of weeks later while visiting Kasey, a mutual HP friend, that Veneeta had a total meltdown after she got off the phone with me. She went to Kasey's office and was so hysterical, that Kasey thought a family member had died. She was sobbing uncontrollably because I had been laid off of my job at HP, and now I had cancer. Since I had previously sent an email to Kasey, letting her know about my diagnosis and my plan to attack it with a sense of humor, she tried to convince Veneeta that I was going to be just fine. Unfortunately, Veneeta was such a wreck, her mascara was jacked, and she had to leave the office for the day.

After I left Kasey's house, I called Veneeta to see how she was doing. By then, she was okay and we laughed about how she was so strong for me on the phone, but crumbled as soon as she hung up. I felt so bad for making her a mess, but it really was all about me at the time.

I started working at Sony on Monday, the week of Thanksgiving. If you can imagine, on day two of employment, I called my boss, Phil Boyle, aside into an empty office to break the news.

"I just wanted to let you know that I have a slight medical condition. I'm going to be okay, I'm going to be fine, but I have breast cancer."

He kept a very stoic look on his face and his eyes subtly started to widen. I rattled on as quickly as possible to deliver the news without interruption.

"I've already had a mastectomy three weeks ago and I feel great. I've already worked two days with no problems. I look healthy, right?"

He slowly nodded as I babbled on.

"I have to start chemo, and radiation, and it starts…tomorrow. I'll come in for three hours in the morning, but my chemo is at 11:00, in Torrey Pines. The good news is that it's Thanksgiving weekend, so I have four days to recover and sleep it off. I'll be back in the office on Monday."

I smiled during the entire delivery of my spiel. I wanted to show him that I was a fighter and a cancer survivor, not a cancer victim. Phil looked at me and very seriously said,

"You do realize that if you don't feel well next week, you can call out sick."

"Yes, but I'm not going to call out. I'll be here on Monday."

"I guess when I go home tonight and work out on my treadmill, I won't complain about my knees," he mumbled somberly.

Perspective, folks. You really have to put your life in perspective. There will always be somebody with worse problems than yours. Life truly is all about how you handle plan B. Accept it, get on with it, and give it all you've got to win.

The night before chemo, my nine-year-old niece, Sara, and 11-year-old nephew, Adam came to visit and brought me the most priceless gifts. Sara sewed a lavender fleece hat for me to wear when I lose my hair, so my head wouldn't get cold. She only began sewing last year when she received a sewing machine for her birthday from her grandma. She's really quite the seamstress and I was thrilled to receive such a soft, beautiful, and useful gift. My sweet nephew, Adam, had sewn a beautiful flannel pillow case, that was so soft and warm. It would keep my face warm while sleeping in the winter months.

On the day I started chemo, my co-worker was explaining to me something that he wanted me to get done that day. (Note that this was day three of my employment with Sony.) I decided I had to tell him about my cancer and that I was leaving early for chemo. I didn't want him to think I was a flake, cutting out of work early on my third day on the job.

What was really cool was that he was very familiar with breast cancer, making it much more comfortable for me to explain my condition as he didn't have as many pre-conceived fears that many others do. He launched into a few stories of his own. As it turned out, his mom had a mastectomy 20 years ago along with chemo. Her chemo made her quite sick because she didn't have the advantage of the anti-nausea drugs available now, but she fared well. She then had a reoccurrence on the other breast about five years ago, and again she came through with flying colors.

Then he proceeded to tell me that he too had breast cancer when he was 20 and had a double mastectomy. I knew men could get breast cancer, but I'd never spoken to someone who had. He then yanked up his shirt to show me his scars. He was very proud of his two measly half inch incisions below each areola, and the quarter inch scars from the drain tubes. I want to emphasize that he still had his nipples and areolas. I thought to myself, that's not a scar...what I had was a badass scar!

When relating this story to my lady friends who have witnessed my lifting my shirt to show off my battle scar, their immediate response was "No, you didn't!" They were right, but damn, my scar was so much longer and more prominent than his. Seven inches from breast bone to armpit, not to mention I have no nipple or areola. I was tempted, but somehow business ethics did not allow a lady to lift her blouse in the office, even when the men could do it. Okay, maybe I could have, but I'd only worked there two days and really didn't want to be fired or have an encounter with human resources so early in my employment.

Cocktail Lounge

I must admit that although I was attacking my condition with positive vibes, I was a bit nervous about day one of chemo. I was back in kindergarten, my first day of school when I was a little bit scared and not quite sure what to expect.

Will the nurse like me? Will she stick a vein the first time or will it take her three or four attempts? Will the drugs make friends with me, or will they make me want to hate them and slap them around?

Sis and I had been preparing for the chemo visits, knowing that they would be several hours. She had gone to all six of her husband's chemo infusions, and they were pretty brutal on Jim. I was determined to get through my treatments in a positive way, and my best friend, Pamela, sealed the deal with her creative chemo kits she prepared for every treatment. She lived in Atlanta, so she couldn't be with me physically for the infusions. The creative kits were the elixir that fueled my upbeat attitude. It was like Christmas morning every time I went to treatment.

For those of you non-crafty folks who don't get why we artistic souls get so consumed with our crafts, bear with me. Crafting is what we do to relax, express our creativity, and to just hang and bond with other creative friends. It also keeps our minds off ugly things like cancer invasions. I would highly recommend to anyone who wanders down chemo lane, to bring a compact hobby with you to the treatment center. Stamping, gluing, and drawing will keep you focused on a fun project so the time passes more quickly.

Sis picked me up from work and drove us to Torrey Pines for the first of many rounds of treatment. I wasn't sure if they're called rounds because they work like Round-up to kill weed invasions, but that thought did cross my mind. I truly believed the rounds would kill my personal patch of crab grass to keep me among the living.

We went first to meet with the oncologist, who explained in detail what to expect during infusions. We opened the chemo craft kit and oohed and aahed at all the fun projects we were going to make. A cross-stitch table runner, a cool star ornament to be stitched and beaded, tags to be stamped (ink pad included), a book that only a one-breasted woman could love, *Lopsided: How Having Breast Cancer Can be Really Distracting,* and pom-poms to celebrate the end of the first treatment.

But my favorite items were two coffee cups from a coffee house in Georgia. The first cup sported the original name Beaner's Coffee, and the second one had their renamed business, Biggby Coffee. Having lived in SoCal my entire life, I couldn't believe that a shop would be named Beaner's, and found it amusing that they finally caught grief for the ethnic slur. Sadly, this slur was very popular when I was a child. No bueno.

For my first chemo, I defiantly wore a white blouse because I have a history of blood spurting from my vein while donating blood. I went into chemo with a Rocky attitude. I would fight like hell to claim victory, no matter what.

The promise of a chemo room with an ocean view was a lie. It turns out that there would be one by next year, but too late for me to enjoy it. Can you imagine enjoying a chemo room? Talk about an oxymoron—cool chemo center...doesn't it conjure up visions of Bali Hai?

In reality, the room was painted a drab beige, and the walls were permeated with a plethora of noxious chemicals. It was tough to maintain my upbeat attitude when the air in the room was almost making me gag. As I surveyed the room, I saw so many sick patients, weak from their infusions, and feeling miserable. I almost felt guilty for being so upbeat, but that was the way I was going to win the battle. I refused to get depressed.

Many of these patients were in hospital beds, sleeping through their eight-hour infusion. I was only going to have a four-hour infusion, so I had it much better than they did. I was a tad worried about the IV since last week the nurse had one hell of a time sticking a vein. But this nurse had her act together. She warmed up my arm with a heating pad for about two minutes, then my veins were popping up as if to get a glimpse of who would be poking them next. She nailed it, and I was on my way. First, Benadryl, followed by two different anti-nausea drugs, and then the good stuff.

During the infusion of Adriamycin, I was given the choice of chewing on ice chips, or a Popsicle, to freeze the inside of my mouth. This drug is so potent, that if you don't freeze your mouth during the infusion, the chemical starts oozing into your salivary glands. At first, I was so nervous that I was jabbering, a lot.

The nurse warned me to keep eating, and all of a sudden I got a putrid dose of the medication seeping into my mouth. It was bitter and tasted like ammonia smells. I panicked and started to wretch and quickly resumed my mouth-freezing. As long as I kept eating the ice, I was okay. It was then that I realized that for me, the smell and taste of chemo would make me puke, not the nausea. For future treatments I always was sure I had a glass of ice water next to me as well. The ice water would shock my system and calm my roiling stomach.

After the Adriamycin was finished, the next drug infused was Cytoxan. Very different sensations occurred during the process and well into the evening. I experienced tingling in my arms, dull pain in my arms, tingling in my head, a headache, tingling in my chest, and very blurred vision. But, the cool thing was that each sensation only lasted about two to three minutes, and then it subsided until the next strange feeling occurred.

Chemo is a good thing. It's killing the cancer. It's not killing me. I will survive!

Sis started working on a star ornament with gold embroidery stitching and we laughed and giggled as she tried to remember how to do the stem stitch. I started on the cross-stitch table runner, but my vision was getting blurry again, so I switched to stamping gift tags. It was fun making different designs, and a bit of a challenge as I was using my left hand, since my right hand was preoccupied with the pesky IV. The nurses loved the tags and thought it was a great distraction during treatment.

The whole treatment lasted three and a half hours, not too bad since I was expecting four. Putting the first treatment behind us, we packed up and headed home. Just as we got on highway 56 heading east, we were greeted by the most beautiful full rainbow that arched across the six-lane highway. Surely it was a sign that all would be well. The cancer drugs would kick butt, and I would be on my way to being healthy again. My positive spirit was uplifted as I prayed a silent, thankful prayer, and peacefully drifted off to sleep.

The fantastic news was that the anti-nausea drugs worked! I wasn't nauseous so far. I had a bonus prescription of Lorazepam, an anti-anxiety drug with the interesting secondary effect of helping with nausea. I took Lorazepam for the next two days as a precaution.

Giving Thanks

I went home and started prepping for Thanksgiving dinner. I made up my pumpkin pie filling, and Denny had his first crack at rolling out pie crust. He did a beautiful job and I taught him how to crimp the crust edge with his fingers and thumb. Denny baked the pie and it looked perfect.

I cooked up the giblets, sausage, onions and celery in preparation for stuffing the bird the next day. I was unsure how I would feel on Thanksgiving, so the top priority was to make the homemade pumpkin pie, followed by pre-cooking ingredients for the turkey stuffing. The rest could be left up to the boys and Denny if I was out of commission.

By the end of the evening I was exhausted, but not nauseous — WOO-FREAKING-HOO! I fell soundly asleep and woke up the next morning fatigued, but not feeling too bad overall.

Thanksgiving was quiet and we had a pleasant day. The boys pitched in and helped with making dinner, dessert and appetizers and we had a fabulous meal. Kyle and Sean made deviled eggs, Sean made a key lime pie, Kyle made a chocolate pie, and Tyler made the stuffing and stuffed the bird. Tyler was also the chief dish washer while I consulted with the other boys making the pies.

It was great to have so much help for a change, as I usually prepared the entire meal myself. I felt pretty good all day, just got a bit tired, and it was easy to sneak in a much needed three-hour nap. I was so thankful for my thoughtful family for helping make this another successful Thanksgiving.

I've always gone out to do the crazy Black Friday shopping, and that year was no exception...with a twist. Donna, my fabulous friend since high school, volunteered to drive me to Torrey Pines for my CAT scan. The scheduler was helpful and scheduled my radioactive injection for 7:30 a.m., so we could hit the early bird sales and be back at the hospital by 10:30 for my scan. By 7:40 we were on our way to the University Town Center (UTC) mall to see what damage we could do.

I hadn't been to UTC in years, so Donna showed me the way to all the cool stores. First, we went to a bakery to have a breakfast sandwich, because lord knows we couldn't shop without nourishment. Fueled up and a cup of coffee under our belts, we hit the mall.

Crate & Barrel, Pottery Barn, and Anthropologie were decorators' delights. We mostly looked, but each bought a little something from Anthropologie. Then, Donna took me to my new favorite clothing store, Chico's! They had such fun and beautiful clothes that I couldn't resist buying myself an outfit. What better way to start my Christmas shopping than with a little something for me! I was anxious for the weather to cool off a bit so I could wear my new faux fur vest, along with the matching slacks and blouse. Plus, there was a bonus of finding a necklace and earrings to match. Voila! Complete outfit. I figured since shopping makes me happy, then that's what was necessary to keep up the positive beat cancer attitude.

Rejuvenated by our shopping extravaganza, we headed back to the hospital for the CT scan. The tech added an iodine contrast to the catheter, in order to obtain a clearer image. I was warned, and it was true, that I immediately had an entire body hot flash as the liquid raced through my veins. What a weird sensation, but after that it was actually relaxing as I closed my blood-shot, itchy eyes and rested for about 20 minutes, while the scanner completed its task.

I headed home to catch a much-needed forty winks. The upside of chemo is that it provided a really credible excuse to take a nap any time I felt like it. Nobody ever questioned me.

Sitting down at my sewing machine, I spent the afternoon finishing a beautiful paper pieced quilt that I started last winter. It was definitely my favorite piece with a cheery cardinal perched on a snowy pine branch. Sewing had been one of my favorite pastimes since I was a little girl, and it was a great distraction from treatment.

I realized that being able to work full-time while undergoing treatment was quite an accomplishment, but my ability to resist the urge to throw up was unbelievably empowering. When the nasty chemo randomly oozed from my sweat glands, I found that taking deep cleansing breaths and guzzling ice water would ward off vomiting.

I knew in my heart that if I threw up even once, it would launch a never-ending downward spiral. I had to beat this, I couldn't cave to the chemo affecting my body. It was so invigorating to know that I could use my mind to overcome my physical state. Yes, I was on to something. I could overpower the drugs and battle the wieldy weed trying to thrive.

I can do this! I can beat cancer! Victory is on the way!

I slept for most of Saturday and Sunday, and as promised, returned to the office on Monday.

True Signs of Chemo

My next three treatments were on Wednesdays as well. As it turned out, this was really great timing for work. I would go home after treatment, sleep for 12 hours, then get up and work a full day. This worked out well for Thursdays and Fridays, although I was totally exhausted by 3:00 p.m. on Friday. It was all I could do to safely drive home after work. There were times when I couldn't even stay awake for dinner at 5:30. I'd fall asleep on the couch because it was comforting to be out where Denny and the boys were, rather than secluded in my bedroom at the north end of the house.

I had the weekends to sleep another 12–14 hours per day. When Monday rolled around, I was feeling pretty good again. Of course, good, was all relative. It meant that I could keep my eyes open for about nine hours, and could fight off nausea with small bits of bland food multiple times a day. Potatoes, Spanish rice with sour cream, oatmeal, crackers, pea soup, and peanut butter were my staples. Fresh fruit gave me sores in my mouth, but applesauce, because it was cooked was okay. Cooked vegetables worked, but not raw, as they, too, would make me break out in sores in my mouth.

Chemo brain – this was the toughest thing to deal with while working full-time, especially at a brand-new job. I became so forgetful, my short-term memory was shot, and on top of it my vision was blurred most of the time. I kept a very detailed notebook with instructions on how to access computer systems. Yes, I broke the cardinal rule of IT and had all of my logons and passwords written down, but I hid them on a variety of pages so it wasn't so obvious. I had names and descriptions of people I met, and even had descriptions of their office location, in case I needed to meet with them. I constantly had to squint, re-focus and enlarge fonts on my 26-inch monitor, in order to read what I was typing.

Just two weeks after my first treatment, I experienced the true signs of chemo. I had been forewarned by doctors and other survivors that three days prior to losing my hair, my head would become very itchy, but it never happened. Thank God I was still able to ward off vomiting, but the hair falling out, not so much.

When I first woke up, I had a burning sensation in my chest, from my armpit to my breast bone, just above my scar. My skin was flaming red, hot, and super tender to the touch. I had an infection and knew I'd be making an emergency trip to the doctor to quickly fight it with an antibiotic. Infections are the number one danger when your immune system is compromised by chemo. A fever over 100.4 would land me in the hospital,

I had no time for hospitals, as I had work to do and needed to be employed to feed my family. Denny was working part time for his shooting club, since his custom home building business came to a screeching halt with the housing market crash.

I rolled out of bed and routinely jumped in the shower. As I was rinsing off, I noticed a huge clump of hair on my leg. What the heck, I thought. Then mumbled to myself, "I guess today is the day." I reached up and grabbed another section of my hair, which promptly came out in my fingertips. There were plenty of areas where it didn't come out, but I wasn't about to go to work looking like a child's well-loved rag doll with ratty hair.

I asked Denny if he would cut off my hair, and he quietly replied, "No." He was really having a hard time coping with my diagnosis and he just couldn't do it. So, what's a girl to do? I got out the scissors and gave myself a haircut. You know, the kind your daughter did when she was about three years old, and you sobbed because she whacked a hunk right where her beautiful bangs used to be. Yep, I chopped, hacked, and cut off everything. If you've never worn a wig before, it's really uncomfortable and itchy if you have hair matted up underneath it, so I fixed that. What the hell, I knew I would see Lucy, my fabulous hairdresser of 20+ years, to have it buzzed into a GI Jane cut after work.

Then I put on my wig, and within thirty seconds, I was looking ever-so-normal with my headful of hair.

Yes, it was my hair. I paid for it didn't I? Everything will be fine. It's just another step forward in beating cancer. I can do this.

I went to work and a couple of people commented on my new haircut. I smiled and politely said "thank you." It would be fun seeing their reaction a month or two down the road when they found out I had been wearing a wig for a while.

The insta-hair was as convenient as a drive-thru. You got what you wanted in a minute or less. I'd highly recommend the drive-thru hair-do, if you wander down chemo lane. It's kind of like the chemo diet where you lose an extra 15 pounds. I wouldn't recommend it to friends, but if you have to go there, look at it as chemo with benefits.

Not only is a wig quick to put on, it's easy to care for as well. My wig was not real hair, but manufactured hair. Once a week all I had to do was wash it in wig shampoo, rinse it out, towel dry, and then hang it out to dry outside. I hung it on a plant stake in one of my potted plants on the deck, because I thought it looked funny and it brought smiles to my boys. Anything to lighten the moment nurtured my goal of happily beating cancer.

The wig gig. I highly recommend it to friends. Especially if you're working at a new company and don't want to freak out others with your beautiful, bald head.

Nurse Ratched Goes for Gold

I called the clinic and made an appointment that morning with the nurse who would check out and treat the infection. I went to see Nurse Ratched, and she clearly did her best to live up to her name. I felt a chill as she entered the room like an arctic wind.

The first nasty words she barked at me were, "Did you cut yourself shaving your arm?"

"No. I did trim the hedge that was getting overgrown, but I used scissors."

"Did you cut yourself?"

She obviously thought I was lying. The truth of the matter was I couldn't even raise my arm high enough to shave under my arm, because my mobility was severely limited from surgery.

"No, I didn't. That was two weeks ago and I have no clue what's going on. The infection just happened overnight."

She said the infection was cellulitis, something that's relatively common, but mostly in men and often in the extremities like the legs. Since this seemed like an odd explanation which certainly didn't describe my situation, I did some research on my own, after I returned home.

Cellulitis can be triggered by several things. Poor circulation in the veins, liver disease, skin disorders, post-surgery, and especially if there is poor drainage in the lymphatic system. Bingo, my drain had been clogged the prior week, and this infection slowly was building in my system, then finally grew to a burning infection. She should have known that since she was the one who tortured me with her reckless drain milking procedure.

"I need to get a sample of the fluid causing the inflammation."

That of course meant another lovely needle to extract the bodily fluids. It really wasn't that bad, but all she got was blood, nothing to culture. In order to withdraw the fluid, she had me put my hand on her shoulder so that she could get a clear shot at where to insert the needle. Because of the infection and swelling, it was all I could do to raise my arm high enough to place my hand on her shoulder.

"You should have much more mobility than this! I'm going to send you to a physical therapist who will really get your arm moving!"

It was all I could do to hold back tears. Here I was in pain, inflamed, drained from chemo, and on the verge of being hospitalized and all she could do was snarl and bark like a rabid dog. I explained to her that I had most of my mobility back prior to the infection, but she was uninterested in my excuse. Not to mention she didn't even notice the cording under my arm, caused by lymph node removal, that was impeding my flexibility.

I glanced around the room to see if there was a bucket I could fill with water, then douse her with it. I would have fun watching her as she melted into a big green puddle. Not a chance. Nurse Ratched would live another day to torture me some more.

She took out a purple marker and marked all around the infection so I could see day-by-day if it improved or worsened. The actual area was about five inches by three inches, just above my scar.

Then she went on to tell me that she was going to give me an injection of Rocephin, and it was really going to be painful.

Thanks, honey. Just what I need is more pain to add to the side effects of chemo and the searing pain in my chest. Bring it on, witch. I'm going to beat this crap come hell or high water.

Nurse Ratched brought in another nurse who started preparing the syringe. She had two vials of medicine, and they were discussing whether they needed to give me two injections because of the amount of the fluid.

"How much do you weigh?"

"115 pounds."

"Oh, then we can get by with one injection and less medication."

Thank God!

Nurse Ratched didn't lie. A 22-gauge needle was not my friend, especially when it was jammed into the top of my thigh (it needed to go into a large muscle and an arm just wouldn't cut it). The other nurse did numb the skin first, but of course that just took care of the initial skin breaking. She plunged the syringe very quickly which made it even worse. Yes, it truly was the most painful shot I've ever had. Hell, an epidural and a spinal tap were nothing compared to this. But wait, there's more. Within five minutes, the pain in my muscle was excruciating. I felt like I had been kicked by a horse.

As a wrap to my miserable appointment, Nurse Ratched asked the standard question, "Are you allergic to any medications?"

"Yes, sulfa and codeine."

She proceeded to write a prescription for an oral antibiotic, which I planned to fill after my trip to the beauty shop for my buzz cut.

I ambled out of the office and had a hard time walking. I hobbled to my car and drove back to work. Because it was about 10:00 a.m., the parking lot was pretty much full and I had to park in the north forty. I was fighting off tears as I finally made it into the building. Thankfully I had ibuprofen waiting patiently at my desk, and popped three of them, which kicked in within a half hour. The real bummer was that I had to go back the next day for another shot in my other leg.

Shifting focus, I limped into the conference room to join my colleagues who were busily working on training slides for the upcoming Consumer Electronics Show (CES). We all were tasked with writing messaging, specifications, and to create informative slide presentations to train our training partners. Focusing on creating informative and interesting presentations was a much-needed distraction to the reality of battling cancer and my throbbing thigh.

Keep smiling. Keep working. Fight on. I will beat this.

After gimping around the office throughout the day, having the rest of my hair buzzed, then waiting in line at the pharmacy for 30 minutes, it was 6:00 p.m. I was exhausted, famished, and cranky. When I finally got my prescription, I read the label, which listed sulfa, one of the two medications to which I'm allergic. So much for taking the much-needed dose that evening. I left the prescription at the pharmacy and got my money back. I was not looking forward to telling Nurse Ratched that I wasn't able to pick up my prescription because of her error.

I went back to see her the next morning for my second dose of Rocephin. When I told her that I didn't get the antibiotic prescription yesterday, she lost it.

"Why didn't you tell me you were allergic to sulfa? When I asked you if you had any allergies, you told me NO!"

"Check your notes, I told you I was allergic to both sulfa and codeine, plus, it's in my records."

"Well, the pharmacy should have called me for a new prescription." She never even apologized for her mistake, and just blamed both me and the pharmacist.

Nurse Ratched brought in another nurse to administer the injection. Fortunately, he used a different technique than the day before. Rather than plunging the needle like a dagger into my thigh, he gently inserted the needle, and administered the injection really slowly, which meant that it wasn't as painful going in. He kept telling me how much of the medicine had been injected, one quarter, one half, three quarters, then done. While calling out the measurements freaked me out at first, at least I knew where I stood, and after 15 seconds the injection was finished.

Nurse Ratched drew a second purple line around the infection, and fortunately, it had receded a bit from yesterday. Rocephin was working. Woo-hoo! She gave me a new prescription and told me if there was any change in the infection for the worse that I had to go immediately to urgent care over the weekend. I needed to keep taking my temperature, and if it elevated to 100.4, I was in deep shit (my words, not hers) and would be admitted to the hospital.

I still had the incredible muscle pain and had a hard time walking, but I took three ibuprofen on the way back to work, which eased the pain. After the ordeal the previous day, I went to the company nurse who gave me a temporary disabled parking pass. Going forward, I would always be able to park near the entrance of the building. It was such a relief to park nearby while dealing with medical issues. I had so many appointments between blood draws, booster shots, chemo, bone scans, and echocardiograms, that disabled parking was one simple pleasure that made my life easier.

Yes, I can do this. This is only a stumbling block. I'm thankful to be alive.

My Adrenaline

On the bright side, when I got home, my new chemo kit from Pamela had arrived. Sis and I would open it at the treatment center on Wednesday. I couldn't wait to see what our new projects would be. The kits were definitely the silver lining to enduring chemo.

On the weekend, my infection had gotten a little bit worse and spread, so I drove myself down to Rancho Bernardo on a Sunday morning, to have it checked out. I'm telling you, Urgent Care is such an oxymoron. It should be renamed to Come hang out with a bunch of sick people for several hours, Claustrophobic waiting rooms are us, or better yet, If you're really sick, lie down on the floor outside the waiting room and we'll take you in. The last one worked beautifully for some lady, who immediately was seen by a doctor.

After more than two hours of sitting in a waiting room with a bunch of coughing, miserable people, I decided it would be better to leave. The receptionist told me it would be another 2–3 hours before I would be seen, and for me, it was much riskier to be around all these airborne germs than to have my infection ignored for a day. Besides, I had an appointment with my oncologist on Wednesday, and she would evaluate the next step.

I'd been heavily warned by survivors and doctors that the side effects of chemo worsen with each treatment. Survivors have the need to share, which is a good thing, but I think they tend to want to scare the hell out of you because that's what happened to them. That could put a damper on my ever-so-upbeat going to kick-this-in-the-ass attitude. But no, I saw it as a challenge to prove them all wrong. Thankfully I was right, and the chemo effects did not worsen.

Wednesday afternoon, Sis picked me up from work, and we drove back to Torrey Pines for round two. When we arrived at the oncologist's office, the first thing we did was open the chemo kit. Just like last time, it was filled with goodies and creative fun. My favorite project was the Christmas Ornaments by Basic Grey. Although those of you who are not into scrapbooking most likely don't know about Basic Grey, it is a line of really cool paper in muted greens, blues, reds, golds, and other colors. That was the same type of paper I used to make my handmade Christmas cards that year.

We were waiting in the room for the doctor, and an intern came in first to check on me and my flaming red infection. She tried to look subtle (although the sour look on her face showed her skepticism that all was well), as she told me it was risky to have chemo with an infection. She left to get my doctor, and Sis and I kept chatting and laughing as we usually did. All of a sudden, Sis noticed that my wig was askew from changing into a designer wrap around examination gown, and told me I looked like Phyllis Diller. Holy cow! I looked into to the mirror, and she was right! It was so wonky! We were both in hysterics.

Dr. Kroener came in and the first thing she said was "It's not too often that I come in a room and hear laughter." That hit me like a ton of bricks. What a challenging job to deal with depressed and oftentimes dying patients who are so forlorn all the time. She had guts to make her career in oncology, and I was so thankful that she did. She was always so upbeat and encouraging, and I knew that she was doing everything in her power to help me eradicate cancer.

She checked out the infection and was pleased that it had improved. She said she was 50/50 about letting me have the chemo treatment, but that my white blood count had improved from 300 on Thursday to 1700 on Monday. We were able to give it a go, but I had to take my temperature every day, and if it spiked to 100.4, I would be heading to the hospital.

She also told me that from now on, while I was taking the harsh chemo, I would get a Neulasta injection a couple of days later. Neulasta is a drug that helps your body make more white blood cells, to help you fend off infection. This designer drug came with a designer price tag of $6,300. Thankfully, insurance picked up most of the tab, except for $80.

Yes, I'm thankful for the insurance that I have. Even though it's $500/month, it covers so many of my medical treatments. I am blessed.

I asked the doctor, "How do people afford this if they don't have insurance?"

Her sobering reply was, "They don't get the drug and have a much higher risk of infection."

As she did the exam, she commented "You really look great. How well did you tolerate chemo the first time?"

"I'm super exhausted and sleep a lot. I've never thrown up, so it hasn't been too bad. Although the chemical smell from chemo is really obnoxious, overall I feel pretty good. It's definitely better than I expected."

"It's great that you haven't lost your hair yet. You must be one of the fortunate ones who won't lose your hair."

"Oh yes I have," I said while pointing to my wig. "This is my purchased hair. Denny didn't even notice that I was wearing a wig, and we chatted over dinner for over 45 minutes. Of course, he is a guy," I said.

"But tell me this, did he notice that you were missing a left breast?"

I totally busted up laughing.

"I don't usually joke around with my patients, but you seem to have a really great sense of humor."

"It works for me. Laughing makes me feel better. Crying is just too negative and depressing."

Yes, for me, staying positive was my adrenalin. My Mary Poppins attitude will take a spoonful of laughter to make chemo go down. And stay down, damn it!

Next up, chemo time. Sis and I went in and set up shop as the nurse prepared my IV for round two. We dug right into the chemo kit and started punching out all the decorative circles to make Christmas ornaments. The nurse kept coming by and checking on our progress. She said it looked like we were having too much fun...and we were.

There was a couple sitting next to us, and the wife was going through chemo for ovarian cancer. She was wearing a really pathetic wig and looked very sad and depressed.

Her husband engaged in a conversation with us and asked "How do you stay so upbeat?"

"Laughter is truly the best medicine for me. The fun distraction of creating projects during infusions keeps my spirits up. Sis and I have a blast creating things, and giving them to the other patients to brighten their day. Does your wife enjoy crafts? She's welcome to join us."

"No, I'm not very creative, but thanks for asking. This must be your first chemo, because you haven't lost your hair yet."

"Actually, this is my second chemo and I have lost my hair. This is my wig."

They both were skeptical. Her husband said "Really? It doesn't look like a wig at all."

"Yes, it really is a wig and it's made from manufactured hair, so it's really easy to wash and wear. Do you want to feel it?"

He came over and gingerly stroked my wig with his fingers. He was beaming as he told his wife, "Honey, it really is a wig. We have to get you one that looks like your real hair."

She was so happy and I excitedly pulled out a Patti's Pearls brochure from my tote bag to give to her. It was such a thrill to bring a ray of sunshine to this fellow chemo patient, by simply recommending a fabulous wig designer.

With this infusion, I didn't get all of the weird sensations of prickling, pain, and throbbing like I did with the first one, so things were looking up. I also was much better about eating a Popsicle continuously to keep my mouth frozen. I was elated that I didn't have Adriamycin oozing into my mouth again.

Yes, I will beat this with a positive attitude, laughter, and fun during treatment. Just say NO to puking.

As we headed home there was no rainbow to greet us, but I was happy that round two was now out of the way, and I was one step closer to being finished and kicking the cancer in the tail. Onward!

At my third round of chemo, when I finished the Popsicle, the horrible chemical taste came oozing into my mouth once again. I've heard patients describe it as metallic, but for me, it's more like a nasty cleaning product. When I started panicking, the nurse brought me some incredibly sour lemon candies to suck on to mask the taste. While it did the trick and overpowered the chemical, my face contorted as I hit an incredibly sour patch. I thought Sis was going to pee her pants, she was laughing so hard at the faces I was making. She did stop shaking long enough to take a great photo.

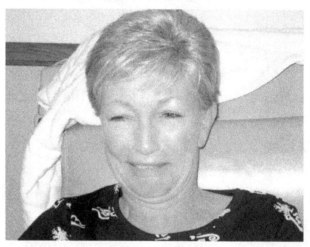
Sour Puss

My favorite project in this chemo kit was the origami lotus flowers. They were really fun and the nurses were wowed. We made them in red, blue, green, yellow pink, and purple. About an hour into chemo, I was getting super sleepy and my vision was totally jacked.

"Sis, you need to put that down. You've been folding the same piece for over five minutes now," Sandra said with a grin.

I put the flower down and closed my eyes for a much-needed nap. Sis then handed the flowers out to the other patients, which brought smiles to their faces. Like I said, fun and chemo. That's what I'm talking about.

A Rainbow of Hope

Thursday morning, I was back to work at Sony. As I met new people at work, I would sketch them, write a description of them, and add them to my office layout map. My chemo brain just wouldn't function well enough to remember all the names and faces of colleagues.

Not to mention, 30-40% of the colleagues were Japanese, so I had to write down their full names. Most of them had come from Tokyo so they had a Japanese first and last name, which was used in their email, but they often took on a different first name, sometimes American, that they would use on their nametag. For example, Hidenori Toyoda, went by Todd. Yosuke Someya went by Somy, and Yosuke Tomoda went by Yo. I had to work with my boss to get all the names and their derivatives sorted out. This really played games with my mushy brain, so it was more of the necessary documentation.

The next Monday, my colleagues returned to the office from the Consumer Electronics Show (CES) where they worked tirelessly each and every January. One colleague returned with a nasty cold. He was coughing and hacking and I panicked.

OMG, if I get sick, I'll end up in the hospital.

Thankfully, Phil, our manager, came in after about 15 minutes and told him he had to go work from home. He objected and said it was just a cold, and he was fine. Phil then pointed at me and said "But she's not. You're putting her at risk for getting really sick. She's a contractor and can't work from home. You can. Go home and don't return until you aren't coughing anymore."

I was so happy that Phil spoke up for me. I had to be so careful at work to avoid any sick people. I would carry napkins and paper towels with me to open every freaking door in the office, and to push elevator buttons. I had hand sanitizer at my desk and used it all day long. The problem with my being stoic and brave was that so many people didn't know what I was going through. If I went to a meeting in a conference room and anyone was sick, I had to move as far away as possible, and sometimes I had to leave the room. This was my pre-coronavirus protection plan, and it worked for me.

At the end of January, I went in for my final dose of Adriamycin and Cytoxan, the two types of chemo I'd been taking for the past three months. The doctor explained that I would move on to a new treatment of Taxol and Herceptin, which would be given every Friday for 12 weeks. She said that hopefully this would go as smoothly as the last three months, but only time would tell.

"Is it possible to move my treatments to Rancho Bernardo? That's only a five-minute drive from work, compared to the 30–40-minute drive to Torrey Pines, depending on traffic."

"Sure. Make it as convenient for you as possible. You'll really like that treatment center which is brand new."

Thankfully, I was able to move those treatments to the closer location. Not only would it be more convenient, the fact that it was brand new meant that it would be fresh smelling not like the current treatment room which was permeated with horrid chemo odors.

Since Valentine's Day was just around the corner, our next chemo kit from Pamela consisted of a fun table centerpiece, Valentine cards with stamps, stickers, and other bling embellishments, along with bright colored markers to fill in extra details on the cards. We dug in and started to put together the centerpiece. It was festive, fun, fabulous, and full of love. The nurses came by to rave about it, so we gave it to them to brighten up the treatment room for other patients.

About 30 minutes into the treatment, an elderly couple in their 80s came in and sat down next to us. The gentleman was there for his first treatment for stomach cancer. He and his wife listened attentively as the nurse informed them of what to expect during and after his infusion. With his IV in place, he glanced over at us as his worried wife fixed her adoring eyes on him. She was so nervous for him, until Sis and I brought some much needed levity to the situation.

He piped up and said "You ladies sure look like you're having fun."

"We are!" we chimed in unison. "We like to have fun and create things to make the time pass more quickly."

Sis grinned and said, "Hey, you don't have any decorations on your cane. Give it to me and I'll make it look really fun for Valentine's Day."

He beamed and his wife started giggling and smiling at him, and then at us. Sis added hearts, X's and O's, kissing frogs, and I Love You candy heart stickers to his cane. It was so much fun to see both his and his wife's attitudes transform from fear to laughing at the chemo that would help him beat cancer. One of the perks of being upbeat during my battle was to share my positive attitude and help other patients. I loved putting a smile on a patient's worried or sad face. I chose to live as a rainbow of hope, instead of a cloud of doom and gloom.

For my first Taxol and Herceptin infusion, I was thrilled to have a very special friend join me at the cocktail lounge. Veronica Glickman was in town for an autism consultation, and she also made time to pay me a visit. I hadn't seen her in several months, and was so excited that she was coming down from San Francisco for the weekend. She was not only going to join me for chemo cocktails, she was also going to bring me an Italian dinner from her favorite restaurant, Fante's. It was such a fun time to visit and chat with her while my veins sucked in the chemo.

When she arrived at the restaurant, John, the owner was just leaving. She told him she wanted to treat me to one of their flavorful dinners, because I was battling cancer. He said he'd be happy to whip up chicken marsala, and eggplant parmesan for us. He generously gave them to her on the house.

Even though my taste buds were compromised, I was excited to eat something different for a change. We sat and chatted and laughed while the chemo did the necessary, but evil task of killing more cancer cells. This was such a delightful way to have fun during chemo. Change it up, and figure what will make you happy to get through the treatments. It worked for me.

One weekend, I was chatting with Kyle about school, his upcoming play, and life in general. With a worried look, Kyle inquired "Mom, can I ask you a question?"

"Sure, buddy, what's up?"

"Does cancer hurt?"

"No sweetie, it doesn't hurt at all. If it hadn't been discovered in the mammogram, I wouldn't have known it was there. It's pretty scary to think how out of control it could have grown."

"But do you feel OK?"

"No, to be honest with you, I feel like crap most of the time."

As his eyes teared up he said "But you never complain."

"I know. I don't complain because I want to fight this positively. If I complain, you'll feel sorry for me and be sad. Then I would feel bad that I made you feel sad. So, I just suck it up and pretend all is well."

"I guess if that's what works for you, I won't worry about it."

"Good," I replied, and gave him a hug.

He warmly hugged me back and said "I'm glad you can fight it like you do."

Me too, buddy. Me too.

One evening in March, Denny was on the phone talking with Mike, his black powder shooting friend of over 30 years. I could tell by Denny's conversation that Mike wasn't doing well with his cancer diagnosis. Plus, Denny was crying, and not trying to motivate him to fight. I told Denny to give me the phone so I could talk to him. I picked up the phone and began challenging and encouraging him to live with cancer, not curl up and die from it.

"Mike, are you going to kick this in the ass?"

Sounding like Eeyore he glumly responded, "Yeah."

I then barked like a drill sergeant, "No, Mike, are you going to kick this in the fucking ASS?"

He perked up and caught my drift. I told him about my attitude and how it got me through chemo.

"I never threw up! I talked myself out of it, took a bunch of deep breaths, chugged ice water, and kept plugging along."

"But all I want to do is shoot my guns."

"So, go shoot them!"

"But I have to do chemo."

"So what? Do chemo, go shoot guns, then take a nap. Actually, take as many naps as you need. Then shoot more guns!"

My upbeat, positive attitude was contagious. He was catching on. By the end of the conversation, Mike was laughing and on his way to fighting cancer. He wasn't going to give up and let it control his life. Mike lived two years after his diagnosis, 21 months longer than the death sentence he was given. He spent most of his free time shooting his assortment of guns at the shooting range with his shooting pals. He didn't give up. My recipe had worked on yet another friend, who although he passed, enjoyed doing what he most loved in life to the bitter end.

In spite of any expectations to the contrary, none of us will leave this world alive. *Carpe diem.*

The Hiccup

When I went in for round seven of chemo, I had a bit of a scary experience. My white blood count was only at 2.1 (should be 4.5 or higher) but the doctor decided to do chemo anyway. I went in as usual, the nurse inserted the IV, then loaded me up with Tylenol, Benadryl, and Emend, followed by Herceptin, and finally Taxol. That particular day, I was the only patient in the infusion room.

I pulled out yet another fun chemo kit from Pamela, and this time it was a bead project to make book thongs — a type of bookmark with decorative string, charms, and beads. I had two of them done and was about ten minutes into the Taxol treatment when I started having difficulty breathing. My throat and esophagus were itchy and started to swell. Denny had just arrived to pick me up and I was starting to panic.

"Get the nurse."

"What's wrong?"

"Just get the nurse!" I was scared and didn't want to waste time explaining to him what was happening. My throat was swelling by the second.

"Why, what's going on?"

"Just get the nurse now!"

He finally hurried off to find the nurse. I was having an allergic reaction to the Taxol, and my breathing was very shallow and almost panting. My blood pressure skyrocketed to 164/102. My lungs felt like they were going to explode. My heart was racing. My eyes were tingling and felt like they were going to pop out. The breathing symptoms were very similar to pneumonia, which I'd been cursed with in the past. The nurse cut off the Taxol, flushed the line, and started giving me Benadryl by IV. Within 10 minutes, I was back to normal and just sleepy. She started the Taxol again but administered the dosage much more slowly, and thankfully my breathing returned to normal.

What was odd was that she was giving me a lower dose of Taxol because my white count was so low. I started racking my brain after I left (as though that's really possible with a mushy chemo brain) and the only thing that was different, other than my low white count, was that I didn't eat lunch before going for the treatment. I would be getting the Neupogen shots for two days following each Taxol treatment from then on, which boosts the white blood count. Hopefully that would prevent any more severe allergic reactions. I also made sure to eat a solid meal prior to the following treatments, to help absorb any side effects from the drug.

All in all, this was the only really bad reaction I had since beginning treatment in November, so I still felt very fortunate. Hell, I was able to get up and work on my blog at 4:00 a.m. Of course, that's only because my sleep schedule was still whacked out, and I was really up at 1:00 a.m. catching up on my reading.

As I continued the 12-week weekly treatments, I was getting more and more used to the routine of the weekly visit for four hours of infusion. I scheduled my weekly chemo treatments for Friday afternoons, which tended to be the least busy day at work. I'd joke about leaving work early for happy hour, and my coworkers seemed amused.

Sis wasn't able to go to the weekly visits with me, as she had to go to work at HP. I still enjoyed the chemo kits, and would excitedly open one prior to each chemo. I'd work on the project of the week, and the nurses would always stop by to see what I had created. Often, I would make greeting cards with positive messages of strength, to give to the other patients. It was such a wonderful feeling to bring a spark of joy to patients immersed in the dismal chemotherapy journey.

Ever since I started the butt-kicking journey, my private road seemed to meander down different paths. Part of the reason for the change in routes, was that the various cartographers had different ideas of the best way to get to the finish line (similar to MapQuest vs. Google Maps — all working toward the same goal, but with different ideas on how to get there). I just hoped they wouldn't lead me to a dead-end road, where the only way to get to my destination was through a grove of eucalyptus trees and a fence.

I was always told that I'd have a mastectomy, followed by chemo, and radiation. What kept changing was the duration of the treatments. First it was four to six months, then it went to 12 months, then 14 months.

There wasn't any change in me physically, it's just that I never got the full story from the oncologist. In hindsight, that was probably a good thing. I'm pretty sure it would have been much more difficult to emulate Mary Poppins, if I knew from the onset that the treatment would be so freaking long. The surgeon, plastic surgeon, and radiation doctor all said I would have four to six months of cocktails – but they weren't the bartender, the oncologist was.

After the 12 weeks of weekly harsh cocktails, I went back to treatments every three weeks with Herceptin, which I jokingly called chemo-lite. Because it didn't affect my vision or make me sleepy, I was then able to bring my laptop to the treatment center and work during infusions. I didn't know of too many coworkers who took their laptops to happy hour so they could finish their work, so I didn't feel guilty at all about skipping out early on a Friday.

Girls Just Wanna Have Fun

I had the most awesome weekend in early April. A friend who was an aspiring professional photographer, came down from Los Angeles to do a photo shoot of me, in all my baldness. Most of the shots were taken outdoors, but we did a few indoors as well with my bike, quilts, and my '32 Chevy. We laughed and giggled like a couple of school girls (of course she was a school girl, as she was taking photography classes at her local college).

Then, on Sunday, we went out to brunch in San Marcos, with another mutual friend who happened to be our kids' elementary school teacher. To top it all off, we went shopping at the Spring Fest street fair in San Marcos. I had decided to go bald again for the day, but as it turns out it was really sunny and 82 degrees, so a white cue ball head was not the brightest decision. I did buy a very stylish sun protective hat, so that I wouldn't fry my head. I was slaying breast cancer, and certainly didn't want to awaken a skin cancer beast.

As we were walking around the street fair, I spied four sheriffs on duty chatting with a couple of fairgoers. One of the sheriffs (turns out he was the sergeant) was just as beautifully bald as I was. I went up to him and asked, "Will you do me a favor?"

"I guess it depends on what it is," he replied.

I whipped off my hat and said, "Since we have the same haircut, can I have my picture taken with you?"

The look on his face was absolutely PRICELESS! He was dumbfounded and couldn't respond. Then he reached over to one of the other sheriffs, plucked off his cap and asked "Will he work for the photo?"

"Nope, he's got a buzz cut and doesn't look like me."

"Well then I guess I can't say no."

The photographer did her thing and snapped a shot of the bald, beautiful, brazen, and very cool looking duo with even cooler looking shades.

All of the photos were beautiful and I loved them all. For me, it was very empowering to feel proud about having my portrait taken bald. The chemo was killing cancer and my hair, but it wasn't killing me!

The Spa

May 27th was finally the day to go to the radiation oncologist and start the process for radiation. Call me crazy, but I was excited about moving on and closing yet another chapter in the cancer saga. I liked being able to check off yet another series of doctors' appointments that are a necessary, but evil process of kicking cancer in the ass.

After being efficiently checked in to radiology, my nurse started asking a few questions.

"When did you have your surgery?"

"That would be November 4th, Election Day."

"And did you have chemo?"

"Yes, I just finished the nasty stuff on May 1st."

"But you're not wearing a wig are you?"

"Yes, I bought this beauty fair and square with real American bucks."

"Oh my god, I've been in this business for over 25 years, and I've never seen a wig that great."

"That's because Patti Joyce is the rocking mama who knows how to make realistic wigs."

My doctor came in next and started asking similar questions.

"When did you have your surgery?"

"Election Day."

"And when did you finish chemo?"

"May 1st."

"But you must be one of them who never loses their hair."

"Nope, this is a wig."

"Wow! It's the most realistic wig I've ever seen."

I'm telling you ladies and gents; Patti Joyce rocks the Casbah. She has fooled many a naysayer with her wig perfection. I would highly recommend her to anyone who needs a wig to cover up hair loss.

In June, I started the new adventure of 33 days of radiation. I told people that I was going to the spa to use the tanning booth. In preparation for the treatments, the technician determined coordinates of the exact area that has to be treated, in order to kill the cancer cells. Then she tattooed me in four spots to mark the coordinates. There were three different areas to be radiated each visit. The timing for each was 27, 84, and 33 seconds. In between each zapping, the technician would come in, change the coordinates and leave the room to start the radiation again. I made it my routine to count down the seconds every time, so I knew exactly when I'd be finished.

While chemo dragged out for 14 months, the most grueling part of my treatment was definitely the radiation. I was told by doctors and many cancer survivors that I might get burned from radiation, but it typically didn't happen until week five or six. Not too bad, I thought. Wrong!

Unfortunately for me, I started burning on day two. It progressively got worse, and more painful, especially by week four. I could actually feel the scorching on my chest as the radiation worked its magic. There was constant burning pain, especially when I applied the aloe vera. But, as soon as the aloe vera was absorbed, my skin felt cooler for at least a little while. I was more than half way through the treatment and thrilled about being on the downhill side.

I'm getting closer and closer to killing cancer. Keep breathing.

At work, I had to apply pure aloe vera gel six to eight times a day. My chest was blistering and peeling on a daily basis, plus the skin was beet red from the burn. This was the time when many more people (ladies only) finally discovered that I had cancer. I would be in the ladies' room applying the gel to my scorched and blistered chest, and then they would notice the burn.

"Oh my god!" one woman shrieked. "What happened to you?"

"I have cancer and am going through radiation right now."

"That's horrible. Does it hurt?"

"Yes, it does. But it's temporary and I just have two weeks to go."

"But you have to tell them to stop! This is really bad!"

My eyes started to well up, and I was trying so hard not to cry. It was so painful and I was doing my best to stay upbeat, but she knocked some much-needed sense into me. I decided to call the doctor to see if he would temporarily revise my treatment plan. I found an empty conference room, locked the door, and started to sob. I was in so much pain and was getting worn out from my battle. I had been successfully holding back the tears for so long, but the flood gates had opened.

No. Don't cry. It will make it worse. I've got to calm down. It will be over soon. Keep breathing.

Fortunately, after about 15 minutes, I was able to get a grip and calm down. The tingling in my arm, numbness in my fingers, and my splitting headache were screaming at me that my blood pressure had gone through the roof. I made a quick trip to the health room to check my blood pressure, and sure enough it was 168/105.

I sneaked out of the office and walked around the block, taking in deep cleansing breaths, and guzzling ice water to calm my blood pressure. The fresh air seemed to work, so I returned to the office to make the call. I re-checked my blood pressure and it was a balmy 128/81.

The radiation routine was to go for treatment at 7:00 a.m. five days a week, in Torrey Pines. On Wednesday mornings, the doctor would see his patients to see how they were doing. This was only Monday, so I was supposed to have two more trips in the fryer before seeing him. When I called the office and spoke to the coordinator, I explained that I was in a lot of pain, severely burned, and needed to see him before continuing with treatments. Her standard reply was, "He only sees his patients on Wednesday."

I quickly retorted with "OK, then I'll see him on Wednesday, but I'm not going to have the Tuesday and Wednesday treatments until after I see him."

She put me on hold and within two minutes came back and told me that he would see me on Tuesday morning to adjust my treatment plan. I'm telling you, you really have to fight for your own well-being and stand up for yourself. For doctors and nurses, it is their daily job and they like to follow a routine schedule, but they will adjust the "normal" routine, if you push them. But you must be aggressive and be your own patient advocate.

I saw the doctor on Tuesday, and thankfully he made a change in treatment plans. He agreed that the repeated scorching and peeling was taking its toll. The next five treatments focused strictly around my scar, and not the huge part of my chest that was flaming red. Aloe vera and Biafine helped, but the doctor also suggested emu oil, which I picked up from the health food store. At $22 an ounce, it wasn't cheap, but I was desperate to try anything to relieve the pain. I tried it when I got home, but it was not for me. It was greasy and difficult to rub into the burned flesh, which made it more painful. It also completely stained the blouse I was wearing, so I tossed it in the trash and went back to using aloe vera.

The rest of week five went better as they radiated another area under my armpit. Six days of no zapping on the original area made a huge difference. No pain for the short duration, and when they went back to that area the following week, it really was only painful on the last two days. Yee Haw! I was done with the freaking spa. I was thrilled to close another chapter in my quest for cancer FREEdom.

Rock Star

In July, 2009, I was hired permanently at Sony. This was exciting news since I obviously proved that I was a hard worker and had a very high level of integrity and dedication. I was able to weather the storm and still get my job done. It felt wonderful to be a real part of another successful consumer electronics company.

Because I had had cancerous lymph nodes removed from under my left arm, that arm couldn't be used for an IV. It was dangerous to have injections, or to overwork the affected arm because it could trigger lymphedema. Lymphedema is severe swelling of the arm and hand due to the elimination of the 12 lymph nodes.

The problem with that was that I had already had so many IVs in my right hand/wrist, that it was getting more and more difficult for the nurses to get a good stick. My veins would collapse, roll, and were just too small to locate at times.

If the IV went into certain veins in the top of my right hand, I could type relatively well. If it hit a nerve, or was in my wrist, my mobility was severely compromised, and I could only use one finger with my right hand. Of course, I could still use all my fingers on my left hand. Very inconvenient, but at least I could be productive and felt like I wasn't missing out too much by leaving the office for a two-hour treatment.

Oftentimes coworkers didn't even know that I had gone for treatment, unless they saw my bandaged hand afterward. I'd simply disappear for a couple of hours, then return to continue working. I even took my cell phone and headset with me, in case I needed to make any phone calls.

In early August I was delighted to have the opportunity to babysit a co-worker's five-year-old daughter. In addition to being adorable, she was quite precocious and so full of energy. When we got home, we played outside with the dog, climbed on rocks, and picked flowers. She even picked a begonia and put it in my hair. After it got dark, we went inside and ate dinner, made a scrapbook, and then made brownies. She was so excited because she said she only knew how to make cookies, and now she would be an expert brownie maker.

We were nearly finished making the brownies (she was in the licking the beater stage) when I had had way too much of the head squeezing wig. I asked her, "Do you know what I usually do at this time of night?"

"No, what do you do?"

"I usually take my hair off, because it's really tight on my head."

"You do?" She squealed and giggled as I yanked off my wig.

"Do you mean I put a flower in your wig? It wasn't your real hair? Wait, put it back on! I have to show your husband!"

She ran out of the room and found Denny.

"You have to come see what your wife can do!"

She proceeded to lead Denny by the hand into the kitchen to show him the magic. He played along and acted totally shocked as I bent down and she yanked off my wig. Endless giggling ensued. And that my friends, is what kept me smiling. Big hugs to this delightful little girl for making my week.

This is a note I sent to a co-worker, the day after he learned that his mom was given 3–6 months to live because of her advanced brain cancer. He was devastated, as anyone would be, and said that his mom was in denial. She couldn't be positive about beating it if she knew it was terminal, he sadly proclaimed. I decided talking to him at the moment wasn't going to work. So, I sent him a note that he could read if he wished, and hoped it would help him fight with her with a smile.

I know you've been devastated by the blow of your mom's cancer situation, but please try to hope for the best. She may very well be trying to beat it with an upbeat attitude, and not just denying it. I know I had several friends and family members declare that I was in denial because I was so upbeat. I really felt that the only chance I had at kicking it in the ass was to take it head on and laugh all the way to victory. Yes, I knew the possibility of death was there, but I refused to let that be what dictated how I chose to live and move forward. I obviously don't know your mom and your family dynamics, but if she is a fighter and wants to fight the beast to the end, try as hard as you can to suck it up and be positive for her. I'm telling you, there were a few times when my friends and family would start the tears and the oh my god you didn't deserve this saga, but I couldn't get sucked into it and let it drag me down.

I wish only the best for your mom, and I hope her fighting spirit will take her through successfully beating this nasty disease.

The next few months of treatment will be trying, but I'm hoping she can weather the storm. Go see her now and use your uncanny sense of humor to help her get through this. She's your mom and is used to being in charge and nurturing the family, but right now she needs you to fight for her as well.

***

One evening in mid-August, a good friend of my boys (and one of my all-time favorite millennials) came over to visit. Mark hadn't been over in about two months, so when I went into the computer room to say hi, he said "Hey, you have hair now!"

"Yep, it's short, but it's growing back."

"But you look really cool. You look like a rock star!"

I loved Mark for saying that. He was always so sweet and always make me feel good. In honor of my Rock Star status, I asked Kyle to take some pics of me with my new 'do.

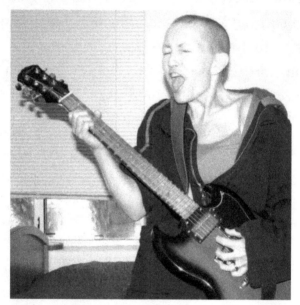

My attempt at singing like a rock star.

I finally got fed up with the wig gig and decided to toss it once and for all. I was taking it off in the parking garage at work, because frankly, I was getting headaches from the pressure dents caused by the elastic. I wasn't wearing it anywhere but at work, and I figured people at work knew me well enough that they could get used to my Annie Lennox look.

My buzz cut made its debut on a Friday. I had the full gamut of reactions from oh my god, you can't walk around the office like that, to wow, you look so fashionable. I did have one woman make a snarky comment saying, "Wow, that's some short haircut."

"Not really" was my sarcastic reply.

"Not really?" she asked with a dumbfounded look on her face.

"No, because technically it's not a haircut if I haven't had hair for nine months."

Yes, she was properly embarrassed, turned beet red, and for a brief moment, I felt bad for her. But she was rude, and should have kept her negative thoughts to herself. I have always been a firm believer that if you can't say something nice, don't say it at all.

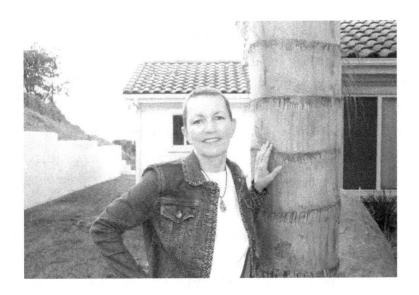

My rock star hair debuts at work.

The rest of the day was pretty amusing to say the least. I got the gamut of looks from averting eyes because I obviously had a cancer hairdo, to WTF, why in the world would anybody cut their hair so short. My favorite reaction was "Wow, you are so totally rock star!"

With the heat wave we'd been having, this was the perfect style imaginable. Plus, my adoring hubby loved it! Or, maybe he just loved the fact that I had hair for the first time in nine months. I've kept my hair short ever since it grew back. The funny thing was that prior to chemo, I never would have dreamed of cutting my hair so short. It was only after it grew back that I realized how stylish it looked.

Survivor Crop

Scrapbooking is a favorite creative hobby of mine. I had been making artful scrapbooks since the 1990s. In 2003, long before my own diagnosis, I started attending a local fundraising event for Susan G. Komen, called Survivor Crop. Survivor Crop was the brain child of John and Camille Akin, the owners of Ever After, a wonderful scrapbooking store in Carlsbad.

Survivor Crop was a one-of-a-kind, 24-hour crafting marathon. Talented and passionate ladies came together to raise money for a very worthy cause, breast cancer patients. The event was always held in October, Breast Cancer Awareness Month.

The ladies, and an occasional gent or two, formed teams called islands. They would choose a clever theme and name for their island. Oftentimes the team would perform a song or dance relative to the theme. Here are a few examples of names that were really fun: Cropping Cuties, Saving Second Base, The Witches of Breastwick, The Wonderful Wizard of Bra's, Booby Bandits, and Save the Hooters.

The participants also all dressed up in costumes, along with decorating their island to represent their theme. There were competitions such as the altered bra contest and shooting marshmallows. All in all, it was a 24-hour wild and crazy event. Survivor Crop was full of creativity, laughter, tears, dancing and inspirational stories of survival, along with the very emotional stories of loss to the disease.

In 2009, I excitedly joined the Survivor Crop Committee to help plan the event. We were in our 8th year and had raised nearly $300,000 for San Diego breast cancer patients. The ladies were chomping at the bit and busy creating island decorations for their islands. We had plenty of contests, games and prizes in store, plus the silent auction, which was always a huge fundraising success.

Our island was called Pink Lemonade, and our team members all got together to design a lemonade stand and cute name tags. We made pink lemons out of clay and added them to our tags. We also had a lemon tree with yellow lemons and one pink one. We won the island decorating contest that year! Our team had a blast and included Sandra, Tanya, Sara, myself, Mayra, and Maria.

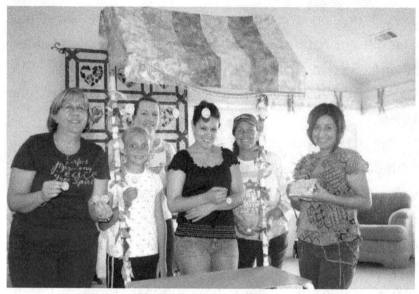

Pink Lemonade stand and island members.

I made a beautiful quilt as an incentive for donations. It was really cool because the winner was my friend, Lillian, who had not only beaten breast cancer, but had also introduced me to Patti, the fabulous wig designer. I was able to raise over $2,800 that year, and our island raised over $6,200. All told, the 129 participants raised over $67,000. It was quite the success!

That was the first year that I entered the Altered Bra Contest at Survivor Crop. It was so much fun to make the bra with a lemon boob. I had too much fun making a mold over the bra, baking it, and then forming the lemon from air dry clay. I added some clear glitter to make it look like a sugar-coated lemon. My boys were cracking up. "Only you, Mom, would make a lemon boob bra," Kyle smirked. I had to keep up with my crazy quest to beat cancer with a wicked sense of humor.

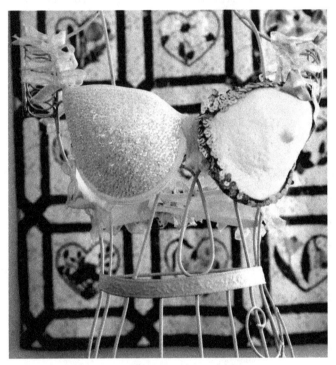

Altered bra contest winner.

I took the bra to both my treatment center and to my oncologist appointments. They were fighting over getting it to display in their offices. Seriously folks, these treatment centers and oncology offices need more than their fair share of levity. It can be such gloom and doom, with all the sick, and often dying, patients. I decided to hit up some of the other ladies who made altered bras to see if they'd donate or lend them to the offices. If they could bring giggles and grins to some of these sick people, I would be thrilled.

By 2013 Survivor Crop had raised over $500,000 for breast cancer patients in San Diego, and we were the number three fundraiser for Komen in San Diego, after the 3-day walk and the Race for the Cure. I was so proud and thrilled to support this amazing event.

Merry Christmas Chemo

One of the amazing things with chemo is the bond you forge with other patients. While most of us showed up for the hook up and got out of there as quickly as possible, there were a few who lit up the room as soon as they walked through the door. One day, my OttLite hero was Mr. Mitchell. While sitting in my comfy chair hooked up to my cocktail lifeline, in pranced the most delightful gentleman, who was in his 70s. He came be-bopping into the treatment center singing Jingle Bells. He took a chair next to me and said, "Good morning beautiful, how are you?"

"I'm just dandy. I'm taking in my cocktails and getting some work done as well. There's no sense letting a pesky IV get in the way."

"You know, this chemo is a good thing. Because without it, we'd be dead."

"You're absolutely right! I am alive!" I shouted with my Rocky victory pose.

It was invigorating to see another courageous soul battling cancer in a positive way. We chatted for a while and then he went back to singing Christmas carols. What a shining star in a potentially gloomy atmosphere.

On Christmas Eve, while most Christmas celebrators were bustling about preparing for Christmas, I had a last-minute pick-up-a-dose-of-chemo-lite moment. Really, it wasn't a big deal, just went into the office to work for three hours, and then headed over to the local lounge to enjoy the holiday spirits.

This happened to be one of the days where the veins on the top of my hand were ornery and uncooperative, so the IV was placed in my wrist, making it nearly impossible to type. I had a deadline to meet and was wrapping up final edits in a Cyber-shot Training Guide, using my right index finger and my left hand to type.

While working feverishly on the guide, my adorable new friend, Mr. Mitchell came strolling in once again. To set the stage, a pro-golfer had recently been "outed" for having an extramarital affair.

Mr. Mitchell, as usual had a smile on his face and a bounce in his step. The nurses were as delighted as I was when he came to visit, as his cheery voice and twinkling eyes made everyone around him feel happy.

"I just came in to see all of my favorite ladies, and to bring you a healthy holiday gift," he exclaimed. He beamed as he presented them a yummy organic fruit basket, and grinned as he read the card aloud. "To all my favorite ladies. Love, Tiger" OMG we all busted up. He was so cute and so proud of himself for making us laugh.

A few minutes later, my phone buzzed, and I saw on caller ID that it was my vendor who would be creating the final print-ready files after my edits were finished. He was in a bit of a panic because he had called the office and I wasn't there. He was afraid I had left for the Christmas holiday break without giving him the edits.

"Where are you?"

"I'm sitting with an IV in treatment and finishing up the guide."

Billy started apologizing profusely and said he was so sorry to bother me. I assured him that he wasn't bothering me and that I worked all the time during treatment. Working kept my mind off the pain from the IV, plus, I was really productive.

I left the treatment center and headed back to the office to tie up a few loose ends. It was a ghost town as only one other person was there. The majority of my colleagues had taken the day off. When I arrived at my desk, my colleague was surprised and asked "What are you doing here?"

"I work here and have a deadline to meet with my training guide."

"I thought you had chemo today."

I showed him my bandaged wrist. "I did, and I worked the whole time. I came to the office first, headed out for a couple of hours on the IV, and was able to finish up with Billy on the phone. Now I'm back to wrap things up and will be done within the hour."

"Well, if it was me and I had chemo, I wouldn't even come into work."

I shook my head and replied with a grin "That's not how I roll. I'm not slacking off just because of treatment. I always meet my deadlines."

The End Is in Sight

One day in January, it was finally getting real. I thought to myself, Oh, my god, I can't believe it! I have 23 down and only one infusion left to go. I really thought that day would never get here, but as it approached, I was overcome with excitement. Excitement for finishing chemo. Excitement for finishing radiation. Excitement for surviving and thriving. Excitement for keeping my job through the whole ordeal. Excitement for having friends and family who stuck by me and put up with my brutal "You have to be positive and no crying allowed" mantra. Excitement for putting this behind me. Woo-freaking-hoo...I was almost there.

I was gearing up for my last chemo-lite treatment, I was trying to figure out what Denny and I could do to celebrate the end of the saga. We've always been huge George Strait fans, but had never been to a concert. I checked out his website, and was so thrilled to see that he had a concert in Phoenix the same day as my last treatment. I contemplated going to treatment then jet setting on a plane, but the timing would have been really tight.

I called the treatment scheduler and asked her to move my treatment up, by a day, to February 4th. This would allow us to take an early flight to Phoenix the next morning, rent a car, check into the hotel, and enjoy a fabulous dinner.

I was so excited the night before the finale. All the perseverance, sucking in the chemo cocktails, and weeks of scorching at the tanning salon were almost over. I survived! I did it! I wrote this poem to express how ecstatic I was at finishing treatment, without throwing up, without crying (well, for the most part), without being depressed, and without missing a full day of work. This was an exhilarating accomplishment, one I wouldn't wish on anyone, but nonetheless something of which I was extremely proud.

Twas The Night Before Chemo Ends

Twas the night before chemo ends and all through the house
Excitement is brewing, I just kissed my spouse.
We're celebrating surviving and not giving in
For cancer I've slain, and I'm able to grin.
There's been surgery and chemo, and tanning salons,

Endless doctors to visit and new wigs to don
But there were numerous positives, I'll list some of them here
Like not shaving my legs and no mascara to smear.
I had fun being crafty with my sis during treatments
With huge thanks to Pamela for all of the chemo kits.
We cut and we glued 'til my crossed eyes got bleary
Then she told me to stop when the drugs made me weary.
When the going gets tough the tough don't give in
So, I hit up an aspiring photographer friend.
She drove into town with her camera and lights
To capture a glimpse of a point in my life
That could have been tortuous depressing and sad
But instead made me feel beautiful, attractive, and glad
That I could be proud of my Charlie Brown head
And kick cancer's ass, and not wind up dead.
So, the end is in sight, a celebration awaits
We're heading to Phoenix to see da-da-da-dah...George Strait
A night much anticipated, we both need some fun
So, wish us well on our adventure, to the Valley of the Sun.

We had a beautiful room at the Hyatt, and the stay was perfect. We enjoyed a romantic dinner at the Compass Arizona Grill, a beautiful revolving restaurant in downtown Phoenix. The views were breathtaking, and the service was outstanding. Our waiter brought us complimentary dessert to celebrate my cancer victory. After dinner we took a leisurely stroll to the concert hall, which was just down the block.

The concert was fabulous. Reba McEntire headlined for George, and she played some of my favorite hits such as "He Gets That from Me" and "The Greatest Man I Never Knew." I was on pins and needles when George came out. He played so many of his hits, such as "Check Yes or No" and "I Saw God Today." But when he sang one of my favorites, "Amarillo by Morning," Denny and I were back on the dance floor on our wedding day, two-stepping to this beautiful song.

Although I was done with treatments, there was the nagging thought in the back of my mind What if it comes back? I'd been harping on my chemo oncologist to get a follow-up MRI but she said it wasn't necessary and insisted everything that had been done wiped out the cancer. Since I was a bit paranoid, I hit up my radiation oncologist and he agreed to order the test. Off I headed to the noise chamber for 15 minutes of claustrophobic fun.

The tech gave me some headphones to listen to blaring country western music to cover up the noise. "You're Gonna Miss This" by Trace Adkins came on during the last two minutes. I was cracking up. OMG – too freaking funny! Yeah, right, give me 14 more months of chemo and 33 days of radiation. It was ever so much fun. At least I have a lot of good stories to tell to entertain my friends and family. I was so grateful for all my family and friends that hung in there with me and honored my demand not to cry.

Joint Pain and Relief

As a preventative measure to ward off the HER2 positive cancer from returning, I started taking anastrozole daily. The plan was to take it for five years. The success rate of non-recurrence was 85% when taking it, so it sounded like the perfect plan.

Unfortunately, one of the side effects of anastrozole can be severe joint paint. The joint pain, similar to arthritis, was intermittent at first, but gradually increased to daily. It affected my fingers, knees, lower back, and elbows. Oftentimes I could work out kinks before getting out of bed in the morning. But other days, I had to continually massage the joints to relieve some of the pain. I ignored it for the most part, but sometimes I had to rely on ibuprofen to get me through the day. It really put a damper on my typing speed at work, and on my bike riding, as it was painful to pedal, brake, and shift gears. I quit cycling because it just wasn't worth the torture.

During my treatment, I had several people suggest that I try medical marijuana for nausea, insomnia, and now, the joint pain. Living in California, we had the benefit of having legalized medical cannabis. Because inhaling any type of smoke made my throat raw, smoking wasn't an option for me, even though smoking a joint for my joints would have been hilarious. I was afraid to try edibles during chemo because any weird taste would make me wretch. But the joint pain was so severe, that I caved and decided to get my medical marijuana card and try it, praying it would work.

I had a good friend who had successfully used cannabis for her medical issues, so I figured I'd give it a shot. It certainly couldn't be worse than all the chemo that was infused for 14 months.

It was amusing when I walked into the doctor's office in downtown San Diego. To set the stage, I went during my lunch break while I was still working for Sony, in a beautiful 11 story architectural wonder of a building. Here I was, a 54-year-old woman in business attire, walking in to get my medical card. The office, if you can call it that, really looked like a shady operation. I felt so out of place. The office was in an old 1930s style home, and clearly they did not use a designer to upgrade it to look like a professional office that I was accustomed to.

Holy cow, the clutter alone was enough to make me cringe. Old 50s café style chairs, a magazine rack from Goodwill, and a coffee table with four year old magazines were in the lobby. The chairs proved to be as uncomfortable as they looked. Two male millennials, bedecked with numerous tattoos and piercings, along with sagging pants, were waiting to meet with the doctor. They both had shocked looks on their faces to see me there. I was pretty sure that they would be making up medical issues to get a card, so they could legally get high.

After the millennials left with their prized letter, I entered the even messier office of the doctor. I explained my ailment due to medication for cancer. She gave me a brief lecture recommending a healthy diet and exercise, then handed me the letter. I assured her that if the joint pain goes away, I would be able to get back to exercising. What a freaking racket. $85 for 5 minutes, and who knows if she was even a doctor. The white coat didn't convince me.

A couple of weeks later, my legal cannabis card-toting friend, Christina, drove me to LA to introduce me to the dispensary protocol. Wow! Capital WOW! This place was locked up tight as Fort Knox. It was an unmarked building, except for the big green cross, that indicated to those in the know, that cannabis was sold there. There was an Addams Family style front door with a small wicket door.

Christina rang the doorbell, and someone from inside opened the wicket door. I was half expecting to hear "You rang?" from Lurch. Didn't happen, but Christina held up her cannabis card and ID, and the door briefly opened so she could go in. I had to wait outside, until she was cleared by security.

Once Christina was cleared, the wicket door opened once more, to peer at this older lady in need of pain relief. Ushered inside, I was greeted by a miniscule waiting room, with a bank-teller type window, bullet-proof window included. The dude behind the counter was built like one of Tony Soprano's thugs. He looked at my medical license and ID, then called someone to open the locked door to the store.

The retail shop looked like it might have been a jewelry store, with the addition of refrigerated and frozen displays, for the edibles. The glass display was filled with very large mason jars, each filled with a different strain/grade of dried buds. The glass shelf was filled with many types of candy bars, lolly pops, tea, lotions, and topical sprays. The refrigerator had a variety of drinks, juices, and home baked goods. Frozen goods had a great variety as well. Along the back wall was a shelf filled with colorful bongs, other smoking paraphernalia, and papers to roll joints. This was definitely a one-stop shop for cannabis lovers.

The owner was a native American man, who really knew his stuff. I explained my situation, and he recommended an edible candy bar to try. I bought the candy, and Christina picked up what she needed for herself, and her mom, who was also battling cancer. The tea worked wonders for her mom's nausea issues.

A couple of days later, I woke up and was getting ready for work. I tried one of the candy bars, by eating a little corner piece. That was certainly not for me. I got higher than a kite, was hallucinating, and it did nothing for the joint pain. I was freaking out! I texted Christina, and she thought it was hilarious. She recommended that I enjoy the high. I didn't enjoy it at all, and threw the candy away.

The next time I went to the dispensary, I told the owner what happened, and he said the sativa strain reacted with my blood pressure medication and is known for causing hallucinations, so I needed to steer clear of edibles with sativa. What he did recommend was a topical spray called ReLeaf, made with the indica strain, and was a CBD product. That spray was a miracle and a god-send. It had no odor, didn't give me any weird reactions, and simply eliminated the pain within 30 seconds.

I used it daily, and it was such a relief that I could type faster and move easier without suffering. I put the spray into an unmarked spray bottle and used it several times a day at work. It cracked me up because nobody ever questioned what it was or why I was using it. I continue to evangelize the benefits any time I hear of someone with chronic pain, such as arthritis.

When the ReLeaf brand no longer could be found, I found another product from CBD For Life. I continue to use it regularly and buy it online.

The Sisterhood

I received a call at work one day in December. It was my sweet friend, Tanya Maurer, whom I worked with for 25 years at HP. She asked if she could meet me by the Sony waterfall for a few minutes. I thought it was an odd request, because usually we would meet to go out to lunch.

As I walked out the front of the building to greet her, I could see that she had lost quite a bit of weight and looked terrific. She had lost 40 pounds since she started Weight Watchers earlier that year. I hugged her and told her how wonderful she looked. Tearing up, she told me she had been diagnosed with late stage lung cancer in late November. She said it had spread to her lymph nodes and adrenal glands. I was the third person she told about her diagnosis. She was very frightened as she broke the news to me.

"They're doing a molecular study and won't have the results until January," she cried. "They said they're going to make me comfortable."

I asked her if she was going to get a second opinion. She said she was told that she didn't need a second opinion. I tried again to encourage her to get a second opinion outside of her medical network, but she insisted that her doctor was really nice and knew what he was doing. I bit my tongue and steered the conversation toward fighting it and beating it with a positive attitude.

We sat outside of Sony headquarters by the calming waterfall and held each other's hand as she spoke of her fears of breaking the news to her daughter that weekend. She said more than anything, whatever happened to her, she wanted to emphasize to Krissy that she wanted her to graduate in June, and pursue her dream of working in fashion in New York City.

By the end of our conversation Tanya was smiling and ready for the challenge. She was determined to stay positive and fight her battle. Each week I would call her a couple of times to see how she was feeling, if she was staying positive, which she was, and to see if there were any new developments.

I last spoke with Tanya on Christmas Day. She had spent the night before Christmas Eve in the hospital, after collapsing at home. She returned home and was spending Christmas day watching movies with her adoring husband, Chris and their daughter, Krissy. She had very labored breathing, but was upbeat and talked of going to see Christmas lights that evening.

The next day she was re-admitted to the hospital. Two days later, Tanya went to her final destination. Free from the burden of cancer, free from all earthly pain. Way too young at 51 and diagnosed way too late. I don't know what the rules of Heaven are, but my plan is to bring her my autographed book that will be dedicated to her.

Tanya has always been an angel on earth, and now she'll forever shine in Heaven. The memory of her beautiful smile, her stunning blue eyes, her zest for life, her true friendship, and her spunky fight to win the battle inspire me and warm my heart. I am blessed to have called her my friend. Love you all and will be praying for your strength to endure and to keep the warm and happy memories of an incredible wife, mother, daughter, and sister alive.

I posted this message on her Caring Bridge site, shortly after she earned her angel wings.

I wasn't able to attend her celebration of life, as I was out of town on a work assignment, but I heard from so many friends about how beautiful and inspiring it was. Many people spoke of fun stories of working with her, and how she was always upbeat and energetic.

***

Because I had been diagnosed with stage three cancer, six months after my annual mammogram, my sister, Sandra told her doctor that she also wanted a mammogram every six months. He was reluctant at first. After she explained how I went from pinhead spots to stage three in six months, he changed his mind and agreed to test her twice a year.

In late spring of 2011 Sis came over to visit. As was her routine, she opened the back door, and shouted "Is anybody home? Then she came down the hall stopped and looked at me and said "Liar." She and I have always thought alike and could finish each other's sentences.

"No! "Do you really have cancer?" I knew exactly why she called me a liar.

"I sure do. So much for you taking the hit for our family." She grinned. "But they caught it really early, stage one. I only have to have a lumpectomy, then radiation. No chemo for me." We high fived.

Her surgery went well and she didn't have to miss much work, just an hour here and there for doctor appointments. When she was in the middle of her third week of radiation, we went to lunch to catch up.

I asked her how her radiation treatment was going and she said really well, and that she only started discoloring and burning the day before. She went on to say that the worst part was the burn on her nipple. Of course, I couldn't that slip by and responded with "Well at least you freaking have one!" OMG we laughed hysterically. Sis said "Only you would put a positive spin on a burning nipple situation."

And that's what I do folks — reality check — put it in perspective. It could always be much worse, so focus on the positive. Onward – Ho!

The Extra Mile

With chemo and radiation out of the way, and my vision improving, it was much easier to focus more on extracurricular work-related activities.

I love being a customer advocate for my company's products, so I would jump at any opportunity to learn and evangelize Sony's wide assortment of electronics.

Operation Musashi was a project where we visited local retailers to make sure Sony products were represented well.

We talked with the salespeople, brought them merchandising items to put on display, and made sure that all the products were in working order. If we found something amiss, we would either fix it on the spot, or call in the support people to fix it for them. We'd give them swag such as pens and pins as a thank you gift. The sales people generally were thrilled with the personal visit, and it invigorated them to sell more Sony products.

In 2011, our charismatic and inspirational president, Phil Molyneux, put out a challenge to all employees to become Master's certified in our online training tool, CyberScholar. It was a part of his initiative, to bring Sony back to booming life to become the number one Consumer Electronics Company in the US.

CyberScholar is a very intensive product training tool with 75 modules, geared to teach sales people about Sony's products. The modules were broken down into product groups; such as TVs, cameras, audio systems, portable electronics, and more. The first five employees to complete the training would win a Project One award of a $500 Sony gift card.

I jumped at the opportunity, powered through the training in my spare time, and earned my first Master's certification. I thought it was a great learning experience, and for the following two years, I became Master's certified again. It really was an effective tool to keep every employee abreast of the products Sony had to offer. And yes, I was one of the Project One award recipients.

I also was asked to participate in a program for our customer experience team to determine how we compared with our competitor's customer's experience. I would purchase and use home theater systems from Samsung, Panasonic, and Sony using the following steps.

1. Purchase the product online
2. Receive, unbox, and verify all content
3. Set up the product and connect all speakers
4. Call Tech Support to connect Netflix online service
5. Test the system to verify that it works
6. Return the product to Sony to break something
7. Take the product home and discover what doesn't work
8. Contact customer service and return the product for repair
9. Set the product up again and make sure it works
10. Write a detailed report of the entire process

Ironically, I quit watching TV back in 1980, so this was a bit of a learning curve for me. I had set up plenty of TVs for demos at trade shows and press events, so that we could playback videos and photo galleries from our cameras. But I had never set up a home theater system, although I'm the chief technology officer in our home, and love to set up electronics. Since these were surround sound systems, I had three sets of wires strung around our family room for the 15 separate speakers, and left them up for the duration of the 2½-month study. My house was a mess, but the study went well, and it was a great learning experience for me and for Sony.

I detailed every step of the way, including documenting conversations with support personnel — whether they could speak English well, could troubleshoot problems, and how quickly the product was returned from repair. It was a fascinating and interesting project and I loved the results. As "payment" for my time, I was allowed to keep the Sony Home Theater System and have the speaker wires installed inside my walls. My testing results were that Samsung provided the best experience overall (like shopping at Nordstrom), Sony came in second, and Panasonic paled in all areas. We had some work to do, and started making improvements.

Because I excelled in my regular job, plus took on many new customer advocacy projects, that year I was awarded the highest performance rating of extraordinary. I was thrilled to be recognized for my contribution and for making a difference for Sony.

Another exciting part of my job was to work industry trade shows to demonstrate and speak about our cool digital imaging products. I specifically worked on point and shoot cameras, which took beautiful photos and videos. In January of 2012, we were launching a set of cameras and camcorders that could shoot not only photos and videos, but could also shoot them in 3D. Now it wasn't just the big boys in the professional arena that could shoot in 3D, but also ordinary customers could shoot 3D to be played back on their 3D TVs.

This was a very exciting time, and I offered to design a couple of visual displays for customers to photograph and video, showcasing the 3D capabilities. I designed two sets of mushroom bogs, three feet by eight feet. I added miniature Smurfs to the set, to tie in with the Smurfs movie that Sony Pictures would debut that summer.

I crafted the mushrooms with mesh, wire, and plaster of Paris, then wrapped them with quilt batting for texture. The first bog was designed and painted with warm earth tones of sage, cornflower blue, daffodil, and tan. The other one was all decked out in psychedelic neon colors.

My colleagues and customers at the show raved about the clever displays, and the 3D photo demos were a huge hit. After that, I was asked to continue making unique displays for trade shows, and each time the theme and design was new and unique. I designed a fall pumpkin patch vignette to demonstrate background defocus — where the object in the front is crisp and clear, while the background is soft and blurred. I also created a barnyard scene with a John Deere toy tractor and a handmade barn. This design was created to show off the partial color feature which converts the photo to bland and white, but only one color such as red, green, blue, or green is visible.

I started incorporating clay sculpting into the vignettes, and would make miniature Sony products such as cameras, tablets, and headphones. These miniatures personalized the displays for Sony, and were a huge hit with customers.

In 2012, Sony had a new claymation movie coming out called *The Pirates! Band of Misfits*. I first made a clay pirate that looked exactly like the main character. I checked with our legal team to see if I could use it at the show. I had to send her a photo of it, then called her to see if I could use it. Her reply was "It's amazing and detailed, but no, because it would be a copyright violation." She explained that an outside company made the characters, so they owned the copyright, not Sony.

Instead, I made a colorful beach scene, complete with my own characters that would imply that it was related to the Pirates movie. The crab, treasure chest, pelican, and toucan, were all designed to once again showcase the partial color effect. I once again received rave reviews about this scene, and was praised for going the extra mile for Sony.

Replacement Parts

When I went on vacation in 2012 to celebrate my brother Jerry's 50th birthday with family, we had a slew of adventures in store. Zip lining, white water rafting, and a dune buggy rendezvous in the desert.

I was excited, yet fearful. Why, because I was freaking worried about losing my breast prosthesis in the river rapids. So, I planned well, wore my bra with a sports bra over it, then tortured my brothers with a grin by making them promise that if the prosthesis escaped and went down river, they would risk their lives to retrieve it for me.

Jerry smirked, had a twinkle in his eye and said "You got it," Robbie cracked up and said, "I'm on," Scott squirmed and nodded because his two younger siblings were game. Sis and I were cracking up because they were nervous and fearful that they'd have to do it. Laugh at the cards life deals you. It really is the cure.

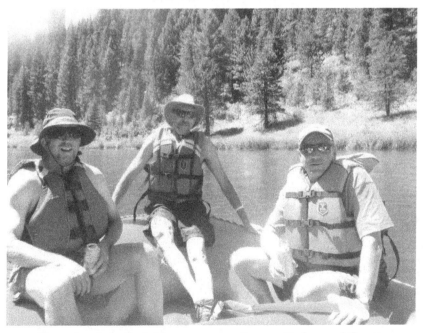

Prosthesis would be rescuers Jerry, Rob, and Scott

I finally made the decision. 2012 would be the year for replacement parts. Four years after my battle began, I tried to ward off panic as I prepared for reconstruction surgery.

Because I was stage three, and had six weeks of radiation, my chest skin was fried. It wasn't pliable enough to stretch to accommodate an implant. I knew the seven incisions, the skin graft from my back, the splicing and wrapping my back muscle to my chest to build a "shelf" for my new implant, would be excruciating. I wasn't looking forward to five days in the hospital and the six-week recovery, but I was looking forward to feeling whole again.

I was sick and tired of not being able to wear the clothes I liked because my chest was concaved. I was fed up not being able to bend over at work to get something out of my desk drawer because someone might get a glance of my scar and navel, as my gaping blouse revealed it.

It was so weird to take off time from work for this surgery, as I never missed a day while going through 14 months of infusions and six weeks of radiation. But it would be very debilitating so I had no choice. I was ready to make it happen and get on with life. I psyched myself up, was a tad nervous, but summoned up Mary Poppins one more time to get through this with a smile. I'd dealt with worse. I could do this too.

As it turned out, the surgery, while quite invasive, really wasn't as bad as I anticipated. Of course, I do have a very high tolerance to pain, so that obviously helped with my recovery and regaining mobility.

The incision on my back was about 8–9 inches long and was more vertical than horizontal, at about a 60º angle. This was to not only splice the latissimus dorsi muscle to wrap onto my chest, but also to harvest a football shaped piece of skin to graft onto my chest for growing and stretching to accommodate the tissue expander.

In addition to the incision on my back, there was another 2.5-inch horizontal incision under my armpit, which was used to tunnel the muscle, blood vessels and skin from my back to my chest, and then the football shaped stitching of the skin grafted onto my chest. I had opted to have a lift done on the right side so that the pair would match, so this involved three more incisions.

Five days in the hospital went by quite quickly. I had an epidural for pain management for the first two days, followed by oxycodone for the following three days. On day two, I was able to get myself out of bed to start walking. My right arm and side were the most functional, so I inched my way onto my right side, then used my elbow, followed by my hand to slowly lift my body up so that I could get out of bed. Painful, but it was not that bad.

I knew from past surgeries that more movement meant more mobility, so I got up and walked two laps around the hospital wing, then went back to my bed to read a book. The next day I walked three laps twice, and by day four I was doing five laps. It felt good to try to get my strength back, but it also was exhausting.

My hospital stay was not bad. The nurses were all very sweet and helpful, and the food was pretty darn good. The only memorable event happened on the last night I was there.

I was reading an awesome government thriller, *The First Counsel*, by Brad Meltzer, and wanted to finish it. I stayed awake until 8:00 p.m. then was so wiped out that I quickly fell fast asleep. I was sound asleep an hour later when two nurses barged into the room, flipped on the lights, and announced, "Sorry to wake you sir, but we're here to take you for your MRI."

I was in a dazed stupor and couldn't figure out why I needed an MRI, not to mention, why they called me sir. They yanked up the railings on my bed, unlocked the wheels, and hurriedly rolled me down the hall to the elevator.

As we entered the elevator, I interrupted and asked, "Why I am having an MRI?"

"Because your doctor ordered it."

"Are you sure you have the right person? I'm from room 417."

One of the nurses looked at her paperwork and said "Oh, we have the wrong room, it's supposed to be 419."

I busted up laughing and they then nervously laughed too.

"I know I have short hair, but I don't think I look like a sir."

We laughed and joked, but I could tell they were really worried about the mistake. I'm sure this is where the fear of medical malpractice lawsuits ensue, but that's not my MO.

I had been forewarned by several nurses prior to my surgery to make sure that each person who was going to work on me checked my wrist band to make sure they had the right person. Now I know why. It would have been funny if they were supposed to do an MRI of male parts. I guess they would have figured it out then, that I was the wrong patient.

I was released from the hospital on the fifth day and it was great to be home. Once the bandages were removed, I could see the severity of the incisions and sutures. Holy moly! I looked like a Frankenstein-ish roadmap. All told there were over 30 inches of incisions. I knew it would look better after time, but it was quite a shock to see all of the red and puffy incisions, and gathered tucks of flesh to re-assemble my back and chest.

I showed one of my best friends, Donna, a week after the surgery, and although she didn't say it, I know she was thinking what the hell were you thinking? I knew it was the right decision for me, and it would just take time to heal.

It was nice to be home with Denny and the boys, and they pitched in to help with whatever I needed. I had forewarned them that I would need help getting out of bed, but as it turned out, I never needed assistance.

My friend who had consulted with me prior to surgery, explained how horrific it was when she had double augmentation. She warned me that it would be two full weeks before I could get out of bed by myself, or open doors. For me, it was simply a matter of always using my right arm to lift myself out of bed or the recliner chair. Two days, not two weeks. Onward and forward.

I quit watching TV when Dallas was all the rage, so it was hard for me to sit and watch movie after movie. It helped that Denny would watch them with me. For the first four days, I watched five movies and one mini-series. Then I moved on to reading another book by Brad Meltzer. I was hooked on his government thrillers.

By the second week at home, I was able to sit and do some hand-stitching of beautiful wool felt Christmas ornaments. Because I had my surgery so well planned out, I purchased the felt and pattern while on vacation in Idaho, and cut them out ahead of time. I simply had to embroider them, then sew them together while recuperating. Very therapeutic, and it kept me docile on the couch.

A month after the first reconstruction surgery, we started the "fill" process on the tissue expander. The expander is similar to a rubber ball, with a metal port. The doctor would locate the port with a magnetic tool, then injected 50cc of saline. Because the grafted skin had no nerves, I initially didn't feel anything but the pressure of the growing expander.

I returned to work the following week and resumed my normal activities. I still had to be careful about lifting anything heavy, and when I worked tradeshows my co-workers did all the lifting and setup, and I would simply work the show and educate our customers about our products.

Every two weeks, for the next three fills, she injected another 50cc. Then on the fifth and sixth, she upped it to 100cc. That's when all hell broke loose in the pain department. Stretching the skin so much quickly radiated the pain all over my chest and into my stomach.

What was I thinking? Yes, I was able to get a new designer breast, but at what expense?

I went in for fill number six, and although it was painful two weeks prior, this time it was excruciatingly over the top. The doctor injected the final 100cc of saline which made me feel like an over-inflated balloon, ready to burst. I left the doctor's office with stretching pains in my chest, armpit, and radiating into my stomach and back. Why in the world was I doing this? Seriously, to have a left chest mound, that was already in place with a prosthesis?

The pain was so excruciating on the way home that I almost pulled off the freeway to call Denny to come pick me up. It would have been smart, because I couldn't even move my left arm, and I couldn't twist my upper body to look over my shoulder for cars on highway 15 as I tried to change lanes. I decided it would be best to stay in the number four lane for the 24-mile drive home. I know I annoyed drivers that were trying to merge onto the freeway, but they just had to maneuver around me.

When I got home, I took 5 mg of oxycodone and went to bed. I woke up the next morning, and the pain in my chest and arm was still excruciating. My left hand was numb and it hurt to breathe. I figured that in another day or two, the pain would subside, so I tried my best to grin and bear it and focused my mind on the future.

When I went to work, I only lasted about four hours. The pain was unbearable and ibuprofen simply wasn't cutting it. I headed home, took another 5 mg of oxycodone, and took a much-needed nap.

As it turned out, the pain droned on for a week and a half. It hurt to take a shower. It hurt to put on clothes. It hurt to drive a car. More deep breathing exercises and positive thinking, and eventually the pain subsided. I still had the phantom daggers of pain that would shoot into my back and arm every so often, but other than that I was feeling OK. I had to go to work, and simply lived on ibuprofen. Oxycodone was too potent and made me dopey and sleepy, so I quit taking it.

Really?

I enthusiastically worked for Sony until the Spring of 2013, when I was laid off, yet again. It's actually an interesting story and I was able to get through the whole ordeal by mentally addressing the challenge with the same approach that I took with cancer. I attacked it head on with humor.

The timing was ironic. When I started working for Sony, I interviewed the day before my biopsy that confirmed I had cancer. I started the job three weeks after my mastectomy, and two days before my first chemo infusion. I was now in the process of wrapping up my cancer saga by finishing my reconstruction. In February, I made an appointment for March to have part two of four reconstruction surgeries for my replacement part.

We all knew layoffs were coming and of course everyone hoped it wouldn't be them, myself included. My boss sent me a meeting request for a one on one, on a Tuesday. When I looked up the room in our Outlook calendar, I could see that the room was reserved all day for human resources. Bingo — I was definitely getting the axe.

Because I had broken the code for the conference rooms, which was unbelievably easy, I was also able to see the names of all the rest of the employees who were getting laid off, including several of my friends. I was the only one from our marketing team affected by the layoff.

I was granted a temporary stay of execution the next morning because for some unknown reason, our department's individual meetings were postponed by a day.

But wait, it got better. The next meeting request I received, for the following day, had the room reserved for me, my boss, HR, and my VP of Marketing. Blackout

Bingo! I was now 200% sure. It was ironic because just two years prior, this same VP had raved about my performance, congratulated me on my extraordinary rating, and said to me "You have no idea what this is going to do for your career." Clearly she was right.

I summoned up my Mary Poppins attitude and decided that this was the swift kick in the ass that I needed to finish this book. It was another gift handed to me. Not a cancer gift, but round two of being laid off. Take the spoonful of sugar to choke down the medicine, and move on to better things.

When the designer corporate headquarter building was built, all of the conference rooms were named after movies or TV shows. It was super fun to see the creativity involved in designing the break rooms and the meeting rooms on each floor of the 11-story building. I found it amusing that they chose the conference room, aptly named Godzilla, to hand out the pink slips — seriously, that was the name of the ghastly movie labeled outside the door. Ironically, if you were called into the 007 room, you were told you had a job. Apparently, James Bond rescued you or something. I guess it didn't make sense to have the layoffs in one of the rooms on my floor such as Wheel of Fortune, Friends, or Cheers. Godzilla? Really? Enough said.

Yes, folks. I really do try to find the humor in everything. It helps soothe the pain of disappointments, and makes me feel like I just ate a Banana Royale from Baskin Robbins. I'm all about celebrating good things.

There is humor in so many life events. You just have to look for it.

I was doing really well and had myself psyched up to use this opportunity to get my book published, until about an hour before the meeting. I had a panic attack and my blood pressure skyrocketed to 179/105. Again, I won't pretend that I wasn't hurt. This lasted for about two minutes until I got a grip, re-evaluated, then chugged down a glass of ice water.

This wasn't cancer, it was losing a job. I would treat the meeting like going to face chemo. It's a step in the right direction.. It will be a good thing. Keep breathing.

I had a slight moment of panic as I opened the door, but the second I saw the manila envelope on the table and the three people with the dreaded looks on their faces, I knew I would attack the meeting with humor.

"Wow," I said, "The manila envelope. That's exactly how I was laid off from HP."

They nervously laughed with me. My boss silently pulled out the chair for me and started giving me the canned sorry to be the bearer of bad news, but the economy is in the dumps, business is not going well, your product is being cannibalized by smartphones, yadda, yadda, yadda, and your job has been eliminated.

Once again, my employer considered me just a number. Get over it. And of course I did.

When the VP talked next, she was incredibly sincere and thanked me for everything I'd done. She raved about my performance and said she had been working tirelessly with other VPs to try to find me another position, but there were none available.

I sincerely thanked her and said, "But this is just the kick in the ass that I needed to finally finish my book."

"What's your book about? Is it something creative?"

"No, I published a creative book back in 2006. This one's about my personal journey of kicking cancer in the ass while working full-time and never calling out sick." The trio's eyes welled up.

"What's the title?"

I beamed and said, "I Shed Two Tears, Then Kicked it With Attitude, which is exactly what I did. I've conquered much bigger challenges than being laid off." More glistening eyes from the Godzilla trio.

I then added with a grin, "But I guess I'll have to rewrite the chapter on Sony." My killing them with kindness and laughter transferred the victim status from me to them. Twisted, I know, but that's how I got through it.

Talk about a whirlwind. I was told I was laid off on Wednesday, and went to a very cool photo shoot the next day at The Mint in Los Angeles. Rising stars, the band members of Walk Off the Earth, were our talent, along with about 25 other local models.

Clearly, the band members had never been to a Sony photo shoot before and were very confused about the process. It was fascinating watching their reactions when they finally realized what was going on.

The story line we were trying to portray, was twenty-somethings going to a live concert and using point-and-shoot cameras to record their experience both in photos and video.

Prior to the actual shoot of them performing live, we were taking all the sample shots which would be used to emulate photos taken at the concert by the fans. We took shots of the crowd outside lining up in front of the venue, the marquee, the fans dancing and taking photos during the mock performance.

We asked them to act like they were performing, but didn't tell them it was just to get the lighting right. Their incredible R.E.V.O album was playing in the background, and we wanted them to simulate performing. We didn't even have their equipment on the stage, so they were warily looking at each other with a WTF look on their collective faces.

Finally, Gianni figured out what we wanted them to do and started singing along with Red Hands. Soon after the others started chiming in. Sarah started singing along with Ryan, Beard Guy Mike, and Joel. After the lighting was set, all the equipment was finally brought on stage, and at last they were playing live.

My colleagues and I were absolutely in awe. They were so amazingly talented and unique, and were well on their way to making it big time. They played all the songs on the album. Our mini concert was a once in a lifetime experience.

At one point, the director handed a Cyber-shot camera to Sarah and asked her to take photos of the crowd. She had fun taking the shots. Then he decided to ask Sarah to crowd surf. She was very skeptical, as were the rest of the band members, because she was six months pregnant with her and Gianni's first child.

All the talent that we had for the crowd, assured her that they would be super careful and not drop her. Thankfully, it was successful and we got the shots we needed for marketing promotions. We wrapped it up, gave them Sony products, and thanked them for their time.

This was the most memorable send-off of my marketing career.

I was back in the office for the next week to pack up my belongings, then headed out to Vegas for a trade show the following week.

Christina and I decided to go for a quiet dinner and reminisce about the good times. I knew that an infectious dose of Christina's hilarious sense of humor would do me good. As we were walking to Wolfgang Puck, Jared, a friend of Christina's asked if he could join us. Jared was such a breath of fresh air, and I really enjoyed getting to know him.

When we entered the restaurant, we bumped into Pulitzer Prize winning photographer, Brian Smith, and his sweet wife Fazia Ali. They both gave me a very warm hug and wished me well. We went to our table and had a wonderful dinner talking and laughing about many topics, none of them included work.

C'est la vie.

Replacement Parts Continued

Five and a half months after my first reconstruction surgery, I was expanded enough to have the permanent implant inserted. The incision would be made on the lower scar from the skin graft, and I would be out of commission for a couple of weeks.

I had planned to work from home since I wouldn't be able to drive, but since I was laid off, my VP told me not to work at all and simply stay home and recover. It sounded good to me, and that's exactly what I did.

I was working on getting psyched up for my next surgery. It would be a piece of cake compared to the last one. The incision would be only four inches long on the new breast, the doctor would remove the expander and replace it with the permanent prosthesis.

The surgery went well and I was only at the outpatient center for about four hours. I was wrapped snugly with tape, pads, and a zip up bra that kept everything together. I came home, took my pain pills, and slept as much as possible. I was dying to see what I really looked like (although I knew it would be horrific right after surgery), but that would have to wait until Friday, at my next doctor's appointment.

This probably sound weird, but I almost wish I had had a double mastectomy. At least the replacement pair would look like identical twins, and not fraternal.

I went to my appointment at 9:30 in the morning on Friday, followed by a career fair at work, and then a final farewell meeting with Phil Molyneux in the afternoon. I was hoping and praying that the hiring companies wouldn't be over the top aggressive with the handshake routine. My chest was still very sore and any yanking or tugging on the stitches would be hard for me to ignore. I seriously needed to keep up the façade of being healthy and perky to try to land a job without wincing. Thankfully, none of the recruiters shook my hand aggressively.

The results from the implant looked better than with the expander, but it was still a little wonky. Odd bulges occur where the fried skin stretched too much or too little. The doctor said this should even out over time. I was fine with whatever the final outcome would be because frankly, I was so done with surgery. I was pretty much back to normal and my clothes fit well once again.

Creating the nipple was another fascinating process of plastic surgery. It's a two-step process and was done in the doctor's office on a Tuesday and a Thursday. She made an incision along the bottom scar of the skin graft that looks like a bird flying with open wings. Then she intricately folded it with her origami skills, and stitched 98 percent of it back together. The body knows that there's been damage, so the blood flow increases. This makes it heal better after step two closes the final two percent.

Wednesday morning, I woke up to discover that significant bleeding began in the early morning hours. The gauze was completely saturated and the Tegaderm Film was bulging with blood. The pressure increased over the next hour, and the blood started flowing out of the bandage. I wasn't in any pain, so I just kept changing the gauze until I could see the doctor when the office opened.

Since I was feeling a bit light headed, I asked my neighbor Karen, to drive me to the office in Del Mar. The doctor was surprised to see so much blood, but by then it had stopped bleeding. She changed the dressing and I had no more problems. The following day, I went in for the final stitching, which was a simple 20-minute procedure.

Five years after I was diagnosed, I went in for the finishing touches on my replacement part. It wasn't a shiny new paint job, but Dr. Arya worked her magic once again to tattoo the areola. My first real tattoo. How cool is that? Most my friends with tattoos were not impressed.

Speaking of tattoos, I had the funniest phone conversation with my brother, Jerry, about three weeks prior to getting the tattoo. I get a kick out of making him squirm with my TMI about procedures, especially since it furthers my crusade of happily beating cancer. I told him I was getting a tattoo to celebrate finishing my cancer saga that began five years earlier.

"Oh, what are you going to get? A cute little pink ribbon?"

"Nope, I'm getting an areola."

"Geez! Do you have to tell me everything?"

"Yep, why should you be different than anyone else?" I giggled.

"You better not show me for real," he snickered.

"Mardi Gras! Check it out bro!"

"I'll throw you some beads!"

Yes, this was another happy and fun moment, thanks to my good sport younger brother.

Once everything had healed nicely, I was happy with the results. The whole process was painful and annoying, but it was also incredibly fascinating. If I had my life to live over again, I would seriously use my artistic skills to become a plastic surgeon. It's such a wonderful art that heals a person's self-esteem, and provides a few more laughable stories.

Mid Life Crisis

The year before my whole cancer adventure began, I took up bicycling. It put my positive spin on my mid-life crisis of turning 50. Instead of having an affair or buying a new sports car, I bought a bike, trained for six months, and then joined my 77-year-old Mom on the ride of a lifetime.

Mom had been cycling since her fifties and always raised money for charities for each ride. Her longest ride ever was from Disneyland to Disney World when she was 64, so she was way more experienced than I. She always wanted one of us five kids to join her on a ride, but we never had the time or desire to do it. So, I decided to take up the challenge and join her in Idaho.

Ride Idaho is an annual bike ride that is not a race. The ride is fully supported and includes meals, drinks, and lodging (tents). Mom had been participating in this ride since its inception in 2005. The route changes each year and in 2007 it started and ended in Coeur d'Alene.

It was challenging, to say the least, and Mom kicked my butt the entire 415 miles. But we laughed, picked wild berries, crashed a time or two, and savored our beer and wine at the end of the exhausting day.

In February 2009, the Amgen Tour of California bicycle race finished in my home town of Escondido. Amgen, the main sponsor, is a pharmaceutical company that engineered two of the powerful drugs that I took to boost my immune system.

The Amgen Tour is the U.S. equivalent to the Tour de France. It is a grueling eight-day race where the riders average 80–100 miles each day. Tens of thousands of people lined the streets for each of the eight stages, to cheer on the riders. Denny hooked me up with Brian Garofalo, a fellow cancer survivor, who got VIP passes for Sis and me to watch the finish up close and personal.

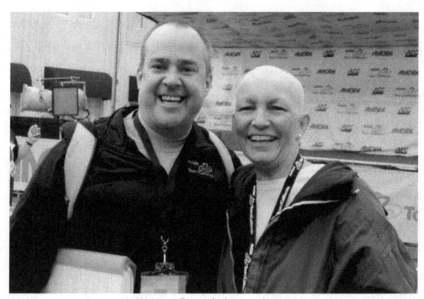

Brian Garafolo and me

The day was filled with fun, festivities, and excitement for the riders. We all hoped that the US team, which included Lance Armstrong, would win. And they did! Sis and I had the most incredible day at the event. The hospitality tent had food, drinks, and the best seats in the house. Everyone was very kind to me as I was sporting my fashionable cue ball look.

One thing that was really cool was a ceremonial ride, called the Breakaway from Cancer Mile, prior to the finish. A local cancer survivor was dubbed the Breakaway from Cancer Champion, and he, along with several family members and friends, led a one-mile bike ride downtown in Escondido.

I vowed that if the bike race ever came through Escondido again, I would do everything in my power to become the Breakaway from Cancer Champion, and lead the ride. I was so thrilled to be fighting and beating cancer with my upbeat attitude, and I wanted to shout it to the world that cancer could be survived.

I was super excited when the Amgen Tour of California bicycle race returned to my home town of Escondido. This time, the race started and finished Stage One in May, 2013. They once again had a contest for cancer patients, advocates, and caregivers to be selected as the Breakaway from Cancer Champion.

My brother, Scott, submitted an entry for me, talking about my whole ordeal and how I kicked it with attitude. He was my family campaign manager, plus I had my friend Regina Hunter from HP, Gini Callahan, Christina Burruss, and Jason Eng from Sony, who all went wild with email and social media. They hit up friends and colleagues around the world, and on April 9th, the last day of the voting and three weeks before being terminated by Sony, I received the email from Amgen telling me that I had won by a landslide, with thousands of votes.

This was such a cool opportunity because I had the opportunity to be interviewed about my experience in front of a large crowd of thousands of people, and it was on national television. Plus, after the race, I presented the Most Courageous Rider jersey to the rider who exemplified courage, sacrifice, and inspiration.

The day of the race was exhilarating. Escondido was alive with excitement. Tens of thousands of cycling fans embraced our city to witness the best of the best competing in America's largest cycling event. It was Mother's Day, and I couldn't think of a better way celebrating with my family and friends, than being at an event that embraced and supported cancer research.

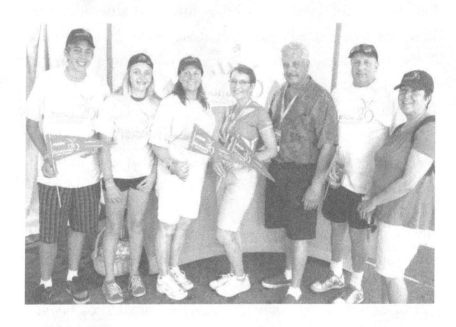

L-R, Adam, Sara, Sandra, Sue, Denny, Scott, and Vienna

I met Bob, a scientist from Amgen and profusely thanked him for what he and his team did to develop specialty drugs to combat cancer. He was thrilled that I was so grateful and said he'd take the message back to his scientists, who get energized by stories of patient's success. Neulasta and Neupogen were two key drugs Amgen developed that helped boost my white blood cell count. I also met Nancy Davenport-Ennis founder and CEO of

National Patient Advocate Foundation, and Rolf Hoffmann, SVP US operations Amgen, both caring people who have dedicated their lives to cancer patients.

I had 22 supporters come join me for the Breakaway Mile walk, including family members, friends, and co-workers. We had a special hospitality tent with plenty of food and drinks, and an up close and personal view of both the start and finish of the race.

After the Breakaway Mile, I was interviewed on stage. When the race finished, I presented the Most Courageous Rider jersey to the winner. All of the people from Amgen were so nice and helpful. What an amazing organization and an even more memorable day.

Inconvenient

How did you do it? I must have been asked that a thousand times over the past decade. I know I'm not the only person who worked full-time during 14 months of treatment, but apparently it was quite the feat. My oncologist was not thrilled that I would put myself at risk by working in a large office environment, but the reality was, I needed a job to keep our family above water financially. This all took place during the Great Recession, so employment was a wonderful thing that not everyone enjoyed.

The distraction of work and taking on a new job with new challenges kept my mind extremely busy and off the pity party path. Did I feel like crap most of the time? You bet I did, but I kept focusing on the positive way that chemo was killing cancer cells. It was not killing me.

If I had to sum up the whole cancer ordeal in one word, it would be INCONVENIENT. The countless doctor appointments, surgeries, blood draws, infusions, booster shots, PET scans, CT scans, MRIs, echocardiograms, bone density scans, and the 33 days in a row 45-minute drive to the coast for radiation, all dragged on FOREVER. I had to work around all these appointments and remain gainfully employed. I think back and am amazed that I pulled it off, but for me, there was no other way to do it. Suck it up, deal with it, work my tail off at work, and sleep as much as possible at home.

Then write a book, to hopefully inspire others to fight their cancer battle, or any other health challenge with an upbeat and winning attitude. Winning is worth the fight.

Being positive and laughing during the journey was my source of strength. The chemo kits were the elixir that sweetened my journey. I encourage anyone who is facing a health crisis to find your own potion, and make it work for you. Stay strong. Fight. Spread Joy.

CPSIA information can be obtained
at www.ICGtesting.com
Printed in the USA
BVHW070947221221
624594BV00012B/1191